# The Story of Cancer
## On Its Nature, Causes, and Control

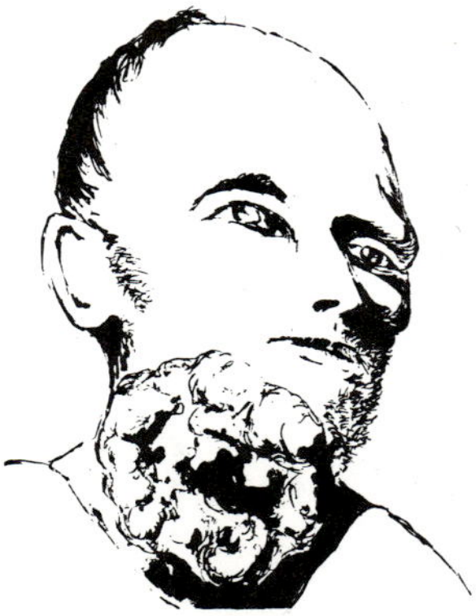

FUNGATING CARCINOMA OF THE NECK IN MAN

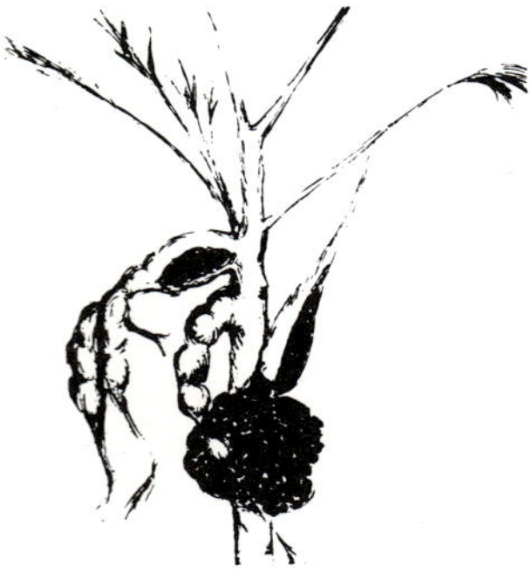

CROWN GALL OF THE PLANT

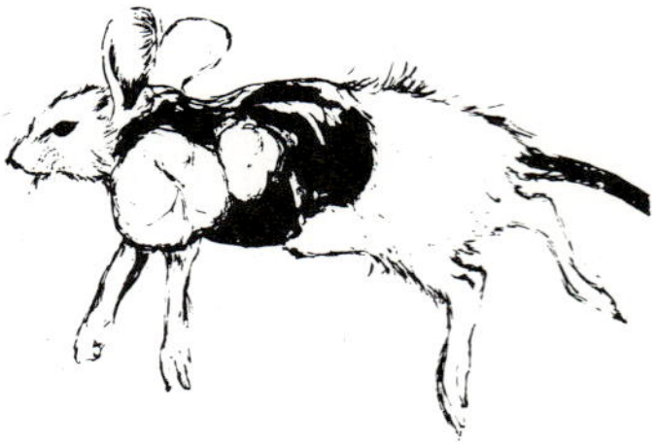

KERATOMA OF THE MOUSE

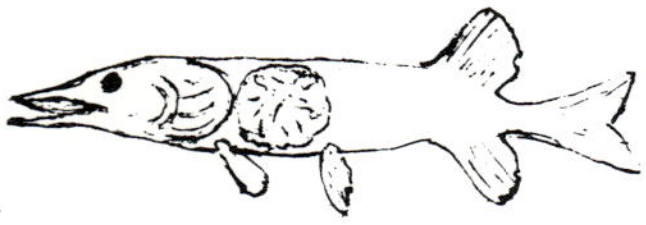

LYMPHOSARCOMA OF THE FISH

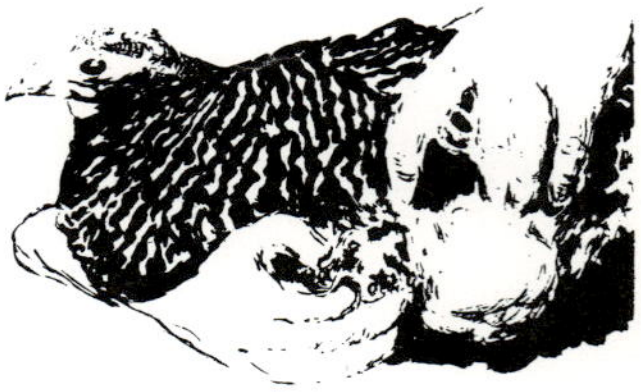

SARCOMA OF THE CHICKEN

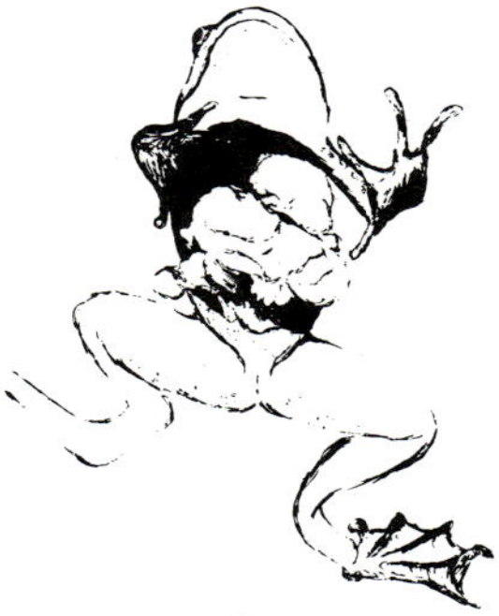

ADENOCARCINOMA OF THE FROG

TRUE TUMORS MAY DEVELOP IN HIGHER ANIMAL AND PLANT SPECIES OF MANY DIFFERENT KINDS AS ILLUSTRATED BY THE SELECT EXAMPLES PICTURED ABOVE

# The Story of Cancer

## On Its Nature, Causes, and Control

**Armin C. Braun**
The Rockefeller University

**1977**
**Addison-Wesley Publishing Company**
Advanced Book Program
Reading, Massachusetts

London · Amsterdam · Don Mills, Ontario · Sydney · Tokyo

**Library of Congress Cataloging in Publication Data**

Braun, Armin C 1911–
The story of cancer.

Bibliography: p.
Includes index.
1. Cancer. I. Title. [DNLM: 1. Neoplasms–
Popular works. QZ201 B824s]
RC262.B67 616.9'94'07 77-13936
ISBN 0-201-00318-X
ISBN 0-201-00319-8 pbk.

ABCDEFGHIJ-HA-7987

Reproduced by Addison-Wesley Publishing Company, Inc., Advanced Book Program, Reading, Massachusetts, from camera-ready copy prepared by the author.



Manufactured in the United States of America

CONTENTS

# PREFACE

This book represents an expanded and more detailed account of four lectures, the Alfred E. Mirsky Christmas Lectures on Science, which were presented by the author at The Rockefeller University to a select group of gifted high school students from the Greater New York metropolitan area. It was the purpose of those lectures to provide not only an overview of the nature of cancer, its causes, treatments, and cures but, more importantly perhaps for students interested in pursuing careers in the biomedical sciences, to illustrate how insight is gained into a complex biological phenomenon such as cancer. Emphasis was placed during the course of the discussion on the importance of selecting appropriate experimental test objects for uncovering fundamental biological concepts that underlie the tumorous state. An attempt was made to show how each in its own way and often because of its own unique characteristics has contributed importantly to our present understanding of the nature of cancer. To provide the necessary background a step-by-step historical account, covering a period of more than 3000 years, of the discoveries and concepts that have led to our present understanding of the cancer problem is presented, as are the essential characteristics that distinguish tumor cells in general and cancer cells in particular from comparable normal cell types. The laws that govern so precisely the growth of all normal cells in an organism are discussed, and an attempt is made to show how those laws are enforced by the organism and why they are violated by tumor cells. This leads to a consideration of the specific substances and cellular control mechanisms that are involved in determining why tumor cells in general grow in an essentially unrestrained manner in their hosts and why, in addition, cancer cells invade and destroy normal tissues and become widely disseminated in their hosts while the growth of all normal cells is precisely regulated. This is followed by an analysis of the nature of the heritable cellular change(s) that underlies the tumorous state and that is ultimately responsible for the abnormal behavior of tumor cells. A point of interest which emerges from this analysis is the demonstration that the cancerous state is not necessarily irreversibly fixed in a cell, as was believed for so many years, but that the genetic information present in many different types of tumor cells can be reprogramed in such a way as to cause them to revert to the normal state. The implication of this finding as it relates not only to the nature of cancer but also to its possible usefulness for opening new avenues of approach for the control of certain cancers is discussed. The methods which are now being used and those which may possibly find future use in the prevention, detection, and treatment of cancer are dealt with briefly in the final chapter of the book.

ARMIN C. BRAUN

# CHAPTER I

# INTRODUCTION

Cancer has sometimes been referred to as "the failure of medicine." This distressing indictment of the biomedical profession is perhaps understandable when it is recognized that of the somewhat more than 200 million people now alive in the United States some 50 million will develop cancer and, of these, some 34 million will die of that disease unless more adequate methods than are now available can be found to cope with that disorder. Yet continued progress is being made not only in the fields of cancer prevention, diagnosis, and treatment but in gaining an understanding of this very complex biomedical phenomenon as well. While surgical procedures, radiation therapy, and the use of anticancer chemicals have in the past and will continue to assist in prolonging life and effecting cures, an understanding of that problem will come only through an application of purely biological approaches since cancer is in its very essence a biological problem of the most fundamental nature.

Before getting into a discussion of our present understanding of cancer it might be profitable to delve briefly into a history of the tumor problem and thus establish the biomedical concepts upon which modern cancer research is based. Such an approach may prove useful because it will serve to illustrate the long and often tortuous path that has been followed to gain insight into a complex biological phenomenon such as cancer. The solving of a problem such as cancer is not unlike putting together a very complex jigsaw puzzle. One must first have all of the pieces and then each piece must be fitted into its proper place if the puzzle is to be successfully completed. In the case of cancer the individual pieces have had to come from work done in many different disciplines and many of the essential discoveries required to understand cancer are so fundamental in nature that they underlie not only cancer but life itself. Thus insight into the nature of cancer has largely paralleled progress that has been made in our understanding of basic living processes.

## HISTORY OF THE TUMOR PROBLEM

The earliest references to what later became known to us as cancer are found in the Ebers Papyrus which was written in Egypt in about 1500 B.C. and which summarized medical knowledge as it was known at that time. Since the first known dissection of the human body was made about 500 B.C. the descriptions of cancer found in the Papyrus were limited largely to superficial swellings and ulcerations that failed to heal and some of these were doubtless cancers as we know them today. By the fourth century B.C., some 1,000 years later, Greek physicians, under the leadership of Hippocrates, had become familiar with cancers such as those found in the breast, stomach, and uterus and it was during this period that Hippocrates assigned the name cancer to these maladies. It is not known why the name cancer (meaning crab) was applied although Oberling (1) has suggested that Hippocrates may have chosen the term because either certain cancers of the breast resemble a crab with claw-like processes buried deep in the living flesh or that the term was used to describe pain similar to that experienced from the bite of a crab. Another 500 years were to pass before the last great physician of antiquity, Galen, who was known to his contemporaries as the brilliant and who settled in Rome in 164 A.D., carried the cancer problem to its next logical step and developed a rather remarkable classification. In that classification Galen recognized what he called tumors according to nature, tumors exceeding nature, and tumors contrary to nature. It was in this last category that all true tumors, both benign and malignant, which will concern us in the present discussion were placed. The word tumor, which comes from the Greek tymbos (a sepulchral mound) and the Latin tumere (to swell), was introduced during that period.

Although nothing really definitive was learned about the nature of cancer during the next more than 1,500 years, diagnostic procedures had by the year 1775 reached a state of sophistication where it was possible for the English physician Percival Pott to correlate the development of a specific cancer with prolonged exposure to a specific environmental factor (2). It was a common practice in England during that period to lower very small boys down chimneys with ropes so that the young lads could sweep and clean the chimneys. This practice resulted in a high incidence of scrotal cancer due to prolonged exposure of the skin to the irritating effects of the soot. This was, then, the first recognized and recorded instance of an occupational cancer due to environmental influences.

Fundamental ideas concerning the nature of cancer were

ushered in late in the 18th and early in the 19th century by the work of the French physiologist and anatomist Marie François Bichat (3). As the result of his studies on human anatomy Bichat recognized 21 different tissue types but, most importantly for purposes of this discussion, described cancer as a tissue although an adventitious and abnormal one. This observation represented a very important step forward since it clearly implied that cancer was a tissue and developed in a manner not entirely unlike that of other tissues of the body.

Although the microscope had been developed much earlier and Robert Hooke in England had published in 1665 in his *Micrographia* the first drawings of cells present in several kinds of plants, more than 150 years were to pass before biologists recognized that cells are the basic unit of structure in all organisms. During the first third of the 19th century rather good microscopes became available. In 1831 Robert Brown in England discovered the cell nucleus and, although he did not recognize its significance, showed that it was a regular feature of all plant cells that he studied. It was not, however, until 1838 during an after-dinner conversation between the German botanist Matthias Schleiden and the zoologist Theodor Schwann that the cell theory in essentially its present form was born. Over cups of coffee following the dinner Schleiden described his studies on the fine structure of plants and Schwann recognized the similarity of the structures found in plants to what he himself had observed in animals. The two men went immediately to Schwann's laboratory where Schwann teased some cells from a developing tadpole of a frog and showed them to the botanist. The two men agreed on the basic similarities of cells found in members of both kingdoms and the cell theory was launched. In his paper entitled "Microscopic Studies on the Correspondence in the Structure and Growth of Animals and Plants" Schwann stated "The great barrier between the animal and vegetable kingdoms, namely, the diversity of ultrastructure, thus disappears" (4). This important concept was not lost to Johannes Müller, who was the mentor not only of Schwann but of a number of other very prominent German biologists and physicians. In 1838 Müller examined under the microscope tumors of different kinds and showed that they, like other parts of an organism, are composed of cells (5). Müller's observation that cancer is cellular has remained to this day the basis of all cancer research.

Although it was known by the 1840s that cells of both plants and animals reproduce themselves by division it was not as yet known that this was the only way that cells could multiply. The theory of spontaneous generation was but one of a number of widely held myths that had served to confuse scientific thought for hundreds of years. Cells were commonly believed to arise spontaneously from formless body fluids such as the lymph as well as from other equally unlikely substances. It was not until 1855 when the great generalization "*omnis cellula e cellula*" (every cell from a cell) was advanced that the problem of cell replication was put on a firm basis. The concept was later expanded to state that cells arise from cells of the same kind and it was finally generalized by Rudolf Virchow, another of Müller's students, to state that all disease, including cancer, is ultimately a disease of cells (6). Some years later Virchow, who was a very capable observer, found that cancers were at times related to chronic inflammation such as is found at the edges of ulcers and fissures, and he proposed that chronic irritation is the cause of cancer.

Since cancer was found to be a disease of cells two possibilities presented themselves. Either the body contains within itself cells that are from the beginning cancerous and the ultimate growth of such cells leads to the development of cancer. This theory was championed by Müller and, later, much more forcibly by the German J.F. Cohnheim who proposed that cancers arose from "embryonic rests" that had been misplaced during the early development of an organism (7). This theory, although widely held for a time and is now known to contain an element of truth, was later largely discarded as being contrary to clinical observations. The second theory, which is now generally accepted, states that any cell in the body that is capable of division can be transformed into a cancer cell.

The next important milestone in the conceptual development of the tumor problem was the demonstration late in the 19th century and early in the 20th century of the transplantability of cancer cells. It was found by Hanau (8) and, independently, by Wehr (9) in Germany and somewhat later by Leo Loeb (10) in this country and by C.O. Jensen (11, 12) in Denmark that when small numbers of cancer cells are implanted into a healthy host of the same species new cancers develop from the implanted cells which are similar in every respect to the cancers from which the cells were originally derived. Cells from the new cancers can again be implanted into new hosts serially over indefinite periods of time. C.O. Jensen showed that this is true not only of animal cancers but it is also true of tumors that arise in plants. On the basis of his studies Jensen stated in 1910 that plant tumors "remind one so much of the malignant tumors in animals that a closer study of the biological relationships of these tumors would undoubtedly be profitable" (13).

The demonstration of the transplantability of tumor cells established the concept of autonomy which refers to the ability of tumor cells to grow in an essentially unrestrained manner in their hosts. The acquisition of a capacity for autonomous growth by tumor cells is the most important single characteristic of such cell types since without it there would be no tumors. Tumors were thus shown to be composed of new types of cells that reproduce true to type and against the growth of which there is no adequate control mechanism in the host in which they are growing. This means that a profound and heritable cellular change has occurred during the conversion of a normal cell to a tumor cell which allows the tumor cell to determine its own activities largely irrespective of the laws that govern so precisely the growth of all normal cells in an organism.

## THE EXPERIMENTAL PRODUCTION OF CANCER

One of the great advances of 20th century cancer research was the experimental production of cancer with the use of specific physical, chemical, and biological agents. During the latter part of the 19th century numerous attempts were made to discover some parasitic organism(s) as the cause of cancer. These attempts were understandable and they logically followed the brilliant successes that had been achieved by bacteriologists in isolating and characterizing the causal agents of many other commonly found diseases of plants, animals, and man. Cancer was attributed at one time or another to almost every conceivable type of microbe but none of the alleged pathogens withstood the critical investigations that are required to establish a causal relationship. By the turn of the present century the parasitic theory of cancer was discarded by all or almost all prominent scientists working in this field. It was during this period that the German zoologist Theodor Boveri proposed the mutation theory for the origin of cancer--a theory that has attracted many adherents to the present day (14). The mutation theory as a possible mechanism for evolutionary change was first proposed by the Dutch botanist Hugo deVries to account for sudden and often profound and heritable changes that he had observed to occur in individual plants during his extensive studies on the evening primrose. Since cancers often appeared to arise suddenly and to involve profound and heritable changes in cell behavior, what could have been more logical than to apply the mutation theory to the origin of a cancer cell?

Although, as indicated above, the parasitic theory of cancer had been largely discarded by the turn of the present century there appeared shortly thereafter several contributions of far-reaching interest. One of these, although not dealing with animal cancer, was published in 1907 by two American plant pathologists, Erwin F. Smith and C.O. Townsend (15). These investigators found that a specific bacterium, now known as *Agrobacterium tumefaciens*, was responsible for the production of a rapidly developing tumorous disease of plants known as the crown gall disease. This finding attracted considerable interest among pathologists generally because at the time of that discovery no animal tumor had as yet been produced experimentally. One year later, in 1908, two Danish pathologists, V. Ellermann and O. Bang (16), showed that a leukemia (a cancer of the blood cells) of the chicken could be transmitted from a diseased to a healthy chicken by means of a cell-free filtrate. Since the type of filters used by these workers precluded passage of organisms as large as bacteria the findings clearly implied that a virus was involved in the causation of this leukemia. In 1910 an American pathologist, Peyton Rous, demonstrated that another malignant tumor of the chicken, in this instance a sarcoma (a solid tumor of the connective tissues), was also transmitted by cell-free filtrates, again implicating a virus (17). The finding that naturally occurring cancers may be caused by viruses represents a very fundamental discovery because, as the British pathologist C.H. Andrewes states, they render "untenable most of the arguments that had been built up to show that the parasitic theory of cancer could not be true" (18). Since approximately 150 different and distinct viruses have now been shown to cause tumors in animals and plants, the virus theory of cancer causation has in recent years received considerable attention and the theory will be considered again later in this discussion.

It had long been recognized that prolonged exposure to strong sunlight and particularly to the ultraviolet region of the spectrum led to the development of certain types of skin cancer in man. This relationship was first recognized in the last century when attention was called to the high incidence of skin cancer among sailors following prolonged exposure to strong sunlight. It was not, however, until 1910-1912 that Clunet and his associates in France reported that they had produced cancers in rats experimentally by application of heavy doses of X rays (19, 20, 21). These investigators described the doses and intervals of treatment required to produce the cancerous growths. Subsequent work done by others not only confirmed the cancer-producing properties of ultraviolet light and X rays but demonstrated that such radioactive substances as radium, plutonium, and other radioactive elements were also effective in inducing the development of cancers. The cancer-producing effects of radiation are perhaps most tragically yet dramatically illustrated in the survivors of the atomic bomb explosions at Hiroshima and Nagasaki in Japan during the Second World War. The incidence of cancers, particularly leukemias, increased very significantly in those survivors who had received considerably less than lethal doses of radiation and who had survived for periods of five to thirteen years following exposure to the radiation.

With the development of the coal tar industry in Germany in the latter half of the last century an abundance of clinical evidence began to accumulate, establishing certain products of that industry as causative agents in cancer. There were reports, for example, of an unusually high incidence of bladder cancers among workers in the aniline dye industry (22). It was not, however, until 1918 that two Japanese investigators, Yamagiwa and Ichikawa, produced cancers experimentally by the patient application over long periods of time of gas works tar on the ears of rabbits (23). By painting the inner surfaces of rabbits' ears every second or third day with the tar for a period approaching a year these workers obtained many tumors and some of these were unquestionably cancers. This work was soon confirmed in other laboratories and in 1933 James Cook and his associates in England isolated 3,4-benzo[a]pyrene from tar, established its structure by chemical studies and showed that it was very effective in producing cancers when painted on the skin of mice (24). From 1,2,5,6-dibenzanthracene, another substance isolated from tar and which in itself was not very effective in producing cancers, a number of highly active cancer-producing derivatives were obtained. Among the most powerful of these was methylcholanthrene which bears a structural relationship to the sterols, bile acids, and sex hormones found normally in higher animals. This compound attracted considerable interest because it was found by Wieland and Dane (25) in Germany that the bile acids can be converted by chemical means into methylcholanthrene. It was thus suggested that cancer-producing hydrocarbons may arise in organisms by the abnormal metabolism of cholesterol, the bile acids, and sex hormones. It has, in fact, now been shown that when human skin is exposed to ultraviolet light a compound with known cancer-producing properties, cholesterol-α-oxide, has been identified among the photoproducts present in skin cells (26). Such naturally occurring substances as the sex hormone estrogen as well as chemical derivatives of that substance have, moreover, been found to elicit a variety of tumors when administered to experimental animals. The aflatoxins, which are also naturally occurring and which are products of metabolism of the fungus *Aspergillus flavus*, have been found to be potent cancer-producing substances. Studies carried out in many laboratories around the world have now shown that numerous organic compounds that range from structurally very simple substances such as urethane (e.g., ethyl carbamate) to the cross-linking agents (e.g., ethylene amine), the alkylating agents [e.g., NN-di(2-chloroethyl)methylamine] to the structurally complex heterocyclic hydrocarbons (e.g., benzo[a]pyrene) found in the tars may cause cancers (see Fig. 1).

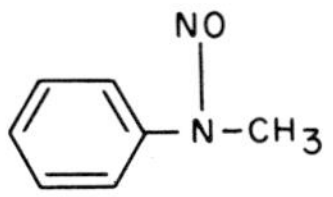


N-Methylnitrosoaniline
(A carcinogenic nitroso compound)

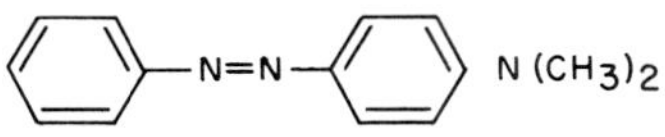


4-Dimethylaminoazobenzene
(A carcinogenic aminoazo dye)

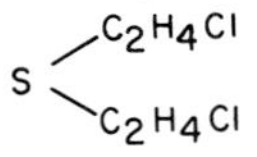


Sulfur mustard
(A carcinogenic alkylating agent)

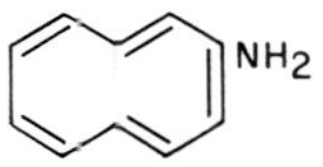


2-Naphthylamine
(A carcinogenic aromatic amine)

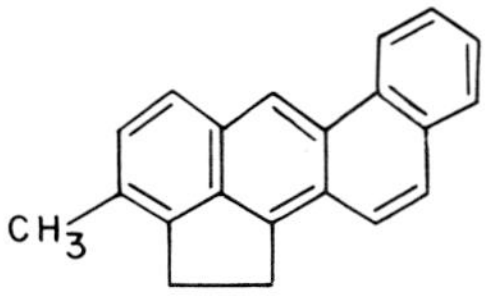


Methylcholanthrene
(A polycyclic aromatic hydrocarbon)

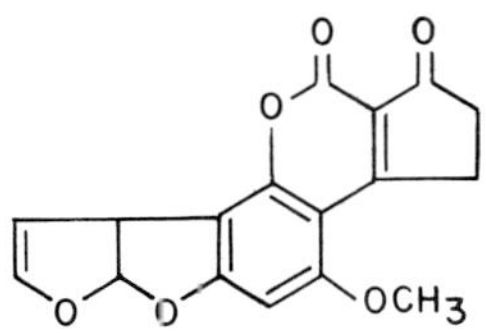


Aflatoxin $B_1$
(A naturally occurring carcinogen)

FIGURE 1. Some representative cancer-producing substances.

Although certain of these chemical substances have been found to be cancer-producing without structural modification many others require structural changes in their molecules before their ultimate active forms are realized. They must be converted by specific enzymes, that may be present in cells, to their cancer-producing form as shown in Figure 2. This change in chemical configuration entails the conversion of a substance to a compound that contains electron-deficient atoms in the molecule which then can react chemically with the electron-rich atoms found in the nucleic acids and proteins

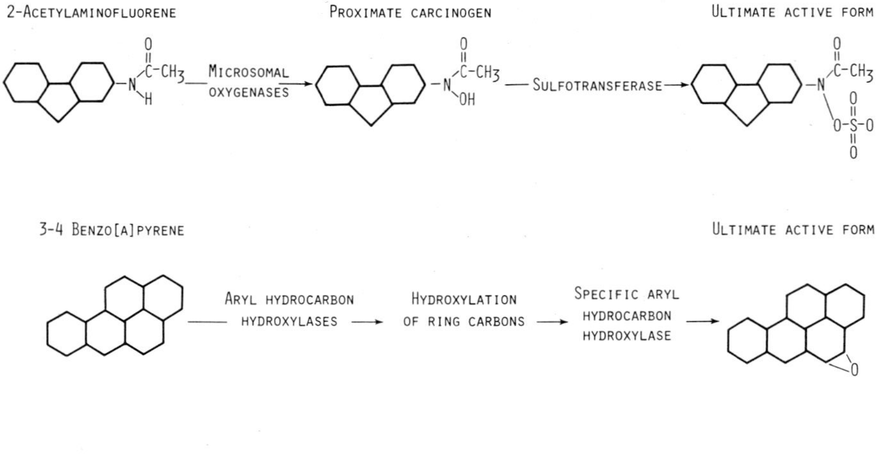


FIGURE 2. Two examples of enzymatic reactions of the type that are required to convert certain cancer-producing chemicals into their ultimate active forms.

of a cell. Whether particular cells become converted into cancer cells would appear to depend then on whether the appropriate enzymes needed to convert a potential cancer-producing substance into its ultimate active form are present in or can be induced in those cells. These findings would appear to be of more than just academic interest because certain studies have shown that approximately nine percent of the white population of the United States has a capacity for the induction of high concentrations of the enzymes needed to convert polycyclic hydrocarbons to their ultimate active forms. Moderate concentrations of these enzymes were found to be inducible in about half the population while low induction rates were found in the rest. It was reported, moreover, that the incidence of lung cancer was about 36 percent higher in cigarette smokers with high enzyme inducibility, about 16 percent higher in those with moderate inducibility than in those individuals who showed low enzyme inducibility in their cells (27). If these findings are substantiated by others it may ultimately be possible to determine in advance those individuals who are most likely to develop lung cancer from smoking cigarettes or from other causes. The results of these studies suggest then that the genetic constitution of a host is a strong determining factor in whether or not a tumor will be initiated. That this is true is evidenced most clearly in the so-called high- and low-incidence lines of inbred strains of mice where in the high-incidence lines virtually every member will develop cancer at a predestined time and even the very tissues or organs in which the cancers develop are commonly predetermined. Some of these inbred lines of mice develop predominantly breast cancers, others lung cancers, while still other lines develop cancers of the white blood cells, etc. These breeding experiments on mice were initiated by the American geneticist Maud Slye (28, 29) who developed a strain of mice which showed a very high incidence of breast cancer and who then proceeded by selective mating to develop a mouse line that was almost free of breast cancer. These findings gave great impetus to later studies on the influence of genetics on the development of cancer. Although humans can obviously not be subjected to similar types of breeding experiments, there is little doubt that heredity plays an important role in the development of certain human cancers as well. For example, a sister of a woman with breast cancer has a three to four times greater risk of developing breast cancer herself than the sister of a woman who has not had breast cancer, while if a grandmother and mother have had breast cancer then the risk of younger females in that family is very much greater than if there were no breast cancer in the family history.

Of the approximately 1,000 different chemical substances that have now been identified as being cancer-producing, a considerable number are found in the environment around us. It has, in fact, now been estimated that 70 percent or more of all cancers that arise in humans are caused by such environmental factors. It is imperative, therefore, that they be identified and removed from the environment insofar as that is possible in modern industrial societies. Prevention is unquestionably the most effective way of dealing with cancer at the present time.

In addition to the numerous organic chemicals that have been found to produce cancer, inorganic substances such as arsenic, asbestos, chromate, cobalt, and nickel-containing compounds have been found to induce cancers. The development of cancers of the lung was found, for example, much more commonly among workers who inhaled dust from chromate ores or those who worked in the asbestos industry than in the general population. Workers in nickel-refining plants developed, on the other hand, cancers of the nasal sinuses.

It has also been found that when plastics of various types are implanted into tissues as films those films evoke the formation of sarcomas (connective tissue tumors) in experimental animals. When these same films are ground into a powder and introduced into an animal in that form they are not cancer-producing. The fact that stainless steel films are also effective in producing cancers suggests that some physical condition rather than a chemical reaction is responsible for the cancerous change in these instances.

Following the development of and subsequent wide use of cell and tissue culture techniques it was found that these techniques provided a powerful tool for studying the tumor problem. Normal cells of many different kinds could be isolated and grown in culture, they could be converted into tumor cells by physical, chemical, and biological agents, and differences in the growth properties of normal and tumor cells could be studied under controlled conditions in culture. It was found very early in the cell culture studies, moreover, that when normal cells of either animals or plants were grown in culture for prolonged periods of time some of those cells became tumorous. This was true despite the fact that no known cancer-producing agent was present in the culture medium.

We are thus confronted with a most perplexing situation. Normal cells may convert spontaneously into tumor cells in culture without the influence of any recognizable cancer-producing agent, the cellular change may be accomplished by physical agents such as radiation, by very simple inorganic and organic substances, by more complex organic molecules, and by very complex biological agents such as the viruses.

All of these agents lead to essentially the same end result. From a clinical point of view nothing distinguishes tumors produced in experimental animals by X rays, cancer-producing chemicals, or by viruses. There is, moreover, reason to believe that in all cases the disease is the same with basically the same underlying heritable cellular change that leads to the development of the cancerous state. If that is true, it would suggest that the underlying heritable change whether initiated by physical, chemical, or biological agents ultimately converges at the same point in a cell. Where, then, could this hypothetical point be?

## THE DEVELOPMENT OF BIOLOGICAL CONCEPTS REQUIRED TO UNDERSTAND CANCER

Before these problems could be approached experimentally by cancer biologists an enormous body of information that was concerned not only with an understanding of the cellular factors and mechanisms that underlie heredity but those that are involved in the regulation of normal growth and development had to become available. This body of information encompasses many of the now well known and classical studies in modern biology and they will be reviewed here again very briefly only because an understanding of the concepts developed in those studies is required as background information for the discussion of the tumor problem that follows.

The fundamental laws of heredity, those of Dominance, Segregation, and Independent Assortment, were, of course, elucidated as the result of studies carried out by the Austrian monk Gregor Johann Mendel, who first reported his findings to the Brünn Natural History Society in 1885. These laws, which were established with the use of the common garden pea, were later shown by others to apply equally well to animals and man. The important point, as far as the present discussion is concerned, is that Mendel's studies showed that most if not all traits that characterize an organism are determined by discrete units of heredity which Mendel called unit characteristics and which we now call genes. The pertinent questions that arose, therefore, were: where in a cell are these particulate elements localized, what is their chemical nature, and how do they exert their effects in determining the specific traits, whether normal or abnormal, that are shown by organisms.

An answer to the first question, namely, where in a cell are particulate elements localized, depended largely on two technical advances one of which was the development and availability of good achromatic microscopes while the second was the use of dyes that permitted the selective staining and characterization of the several distinct organelles present in a cell. With the availability of both in the last half of the 19th century the nucleus was shown with very few exceptions to be a characteristic feature of cells. These methods also revealed the transient appearance of rod-shaped structures, which we now call chromosomes, and which appeared in the nucleus shortly before it divided into two. The chromosomes were observed to split lengthwise and each member of a pair was seen to be drawn to opposite ends of a cell before the cell divided. Here then was a plausible mechanism by which the genetic information present in a cell was partitioned equally between the two daughter cells and the chromosomal theory of heredity was born. This theory received further support when it was found that all cells, except the gametes or sex cells, within a given species of animal or plant characteristically contain the same number of chromosomes. The sperm and egg cells were found to contain half that number.

With this information in hand the American zoologist Thomas Hunt Morgan and his students greatly expanded our insight into the mechanisms underlying heredity. Using the common fruit fly *Drosophila* as their experimental test object these workers brilliantly demonstrated not only that individual genes were lined up along the long axes of the chromosomes but their experimental methods had become so sophisticated that they were able to map the chromosomes and determine the precise location of specific genes on the chromosomes. These studies were greatly facilitated by the demonstration by H.J. Muller, a student of Morgan, that X-irradiation of sperm cells of the insect was highly effective in producing mutations since mutations of specific genes were important markers used by members of this group to map the chromosomes (30).

Having firmly established the fact that specific genes determine specific traits of an organism and that the genes were located on the chromosomes, the pertinent question that arose next was precisely how the genes exert their effects as determiners of hereditary traits. This question was resolved in 1940 when two American scientists, George Beadle, a geneticist, and Edward Tatum, a biochemist, combined their talents and provided excellent experimental evidence for the so-called one gene-one enzyme hypothesis or, as it was later known, the one gene-one polypeptide theory since not all proteins are enzymes (31). Working with the lower plant species, the common bread mold Neurospora crassa, these investigators irradiated the fungus with X rays, as Muller had done earlier with the fruit fly, to obtain mutant forms of that organism. Many of these mutant forms did not grow on a basic culture medium that supported excellent growth of the wild type unirradiated form from which the mutants had been derived. It was found, however, that when the basic culture medium was supplemented with a specific amino acid, a specific vitamin or other essential growth factor, depending on the nature of the mutation, growth of the mutant form occurred. This meant very simply that the mutant form had lost the ability to manufacture a specific substance required for growth. That is, when a particular gene was damaged by X-irradiation or by other means a specific protein needed to produce the specific substance was not made by the cell.

By the time that the Beadle and Tatum work was published a great deal had been learned about the specific metabolic processes by which cells maintain themselves and grow. All of the essential amino acids, the building blocks from which proteins are made, had been characterized. Several hundred different and distinct enzymes had been identified and some of these had been isolated in pure form and shown to be proteins. The great specificity of enzyme action in catalyzing chemical reactions in a cell had been recognized and the central role that enzymes play in controlling cellular metabolism had become clear. Most of the vitamins, hormones, and essential metabolites had been identified and the role that each of these plays in maintaining a living organism had in broad outline been elucidated. Yet nothing was known at that time about the chemical nature of the gene. Insight into this question was obtained in 1944 when three American scientists, Oswald Avery, Colin MacLeod, and Maclyn McCarty, isolated and identified the biologically active material (32). In 1928 the British bacteriologist Fred Griffith, working with the pneumococcus, the causal bacterium of pneumococcal pneumonia of humans, found quite by accident that a specific trait, that of the ability to produce a capsule which forms the outer coat of that bacterium, could be transmitted from a strain of the bacterium that possessed the ability to form the capsule to a strain that had lost that ability (33). Once that trait had been acquired by the normally noncapsule-forming strain it was transmitted as a heritable cellular trait to the progeny of the bacterium. This as yet uncharacterized substance thus behaved like a gene. Using this very simple marker of capsule formation in the pneumococcus Avery and his coworkers isolated the specific substance that transmitted the specific trait from a capsule-producing strain of the bacterium to the noncapsule-forming strain and showed it to be deoxyribonucleic acid (DNA). This very substance had ironically been isolated and in part characterized chemically by the Swiss chemist Frederick Miescher as early as 1869, first from human pus cells and later from salmon sperm, but the central role that it was to play in biology remained obscure for more than 70 years. Prior to the discovery of the biological role of DNA the chemistry of not only that substance but another type of nucleic acid known as ribonucleic acid (RNA) had been studied. DNA was found to contain four bases two of which, adenine and guanine, were purines while the other two, thymine and cytosine, were pyrimidines. Each of these bases was found to contain a phosphate group and a deoxyribose sugar molecule when present in a DNA molecule. When these two components are present on the bases the compounds are known as nucleotides. The other class of nucleic acids, the ribonucleic acids, differed from DNA in that uracil was found in place of thymine and the sugar was ribose instead of deoxyribose. A most important contribution to our understanding of the molecular structure of the DNA molecule came from the finding of the American biochemist Erwin Chargaff who reported that an equivalent amount of adenine and thymine, on the one hand, and guanine and cytosine, on the other, were present in the DNA molecule. This suggested that the bases were paired in that molecule (34). Meantime, studies of the DNA molecule carried out in England by H.K. Wilkins and his associates (35) and Rosalind Franklin and her collaborator (36) with a technique known as X-ray crystallography suggested that the DNA molecule was present in cells in the form of a helix and that the helix completed one turn for every ten nucleotides in the molecule. These studies also suggested that differences in the genetic role of DNA must be in the order of the nucleotides present in the molecule rather than in the gross structure of the molecule as such. With this information in hand the American James Watson and the Englishman Francis Crick brilliantly devised the now celebrated double helix model for the DNA molecule which accounted both for its ability to be copied in the form of a complementary DNA strand as well as for an ability to replicate itself, both of which are essential to account for genetic continuity shown by DNA present in a living organism (37, 38). This theoretical model was found to be correct by subsequent experimental work which demonstrated that the two DNA strands of the helix retain their integrity between cell divisions, as would be expected if they did, in fact, convey genetic information to the daughter cells. The total structure of a specific bacterial gene has been determined by H. Gobind Khorana and his associates in this country (39). This specific gene has now been synthesized in the laboratory and when the artificially produced gene was introduced into appropriate bacteria it was found to be fully functional, thus providing the ultimate proof that the theoretical considerations upon which DNA genetics is based are correct.

A most important step in the development of the problem

of gene function was concerned with the mechanism by which the genetic information present in a gene is first transcribed and later translated into a specific protein. Here, very briefly, it was found that the DNA of the gene is transcribed in the form of a complementary copy of RNA which is known as messenger or mRNA since it contains the DNA message. This mRNA then moves out of the nucleus and into the cytoplasm of a cell and attaches itself to small RNA-protein-containing particles that are known as ribosomes. It is on the ribosomal-attached mRNA that the new protein is synthesized. The question that remained, however, was how are the essential amino acids that make up the specific protein placed in their proper sequence during the synthesis of the protein in a cell. This problem was resolved when a third type of RNA, which is relatively small and which became known as transfer or tRNA, was discovered. The tRNA, like mRNA and ribosomal RNA, is specified genetically. The tRNA carries the amino acids necessary for protein synthesis to the mRNA attached to ribosomes. The amino acids are then arranged linearly one by one on the mRNA template and the amino acids are joined together through peptide linkages until the new protein is synthesized. The correct lining up of the amino acids on the mRNA for the synthesis of a specific protein is made possible because of a four-letter alphabet corresponding to the four bases found in DNA. Crick and his associates in England suggested that a three-letter code could provide 20 clear alternatives required for the incorporation of 20 essential amino acids into enzymes and other proteins and thus provide a non-overlapping code (40).

The American biochemist Marshall Nirenberg and his associate J.H. Matthaei deciphered the genetic code just 17 years after Avery and his coworkers had shown DNA to be the carrier of genetic information in a cell. By mixing in a test tube ribosomes, specific enzymes, an energy source, and radioactive amino acids together with a small synthetic polymer which contained only uracil (poly U) as the base, it was found that only the amino acid phenylalanine was incorporated into the peptide that was synthesized. Thus UUU coded for phenylalanine. It was found that other triplets such as, for example, AUU coded for tyrosine, AGU for methionine, GGU for tryptophan (41), etc. It soon became apparent, however, that more than one permutation of bases could code for the same amino acid and thus CGG, GCG, and GGC all coded for glycine while, for example, CCU, CUC, and UCC were found to code for both proline and serine. The genetic code was thus overlapping and degenerate. While the finding of an overlapping code initially caused concern, subsequent studies carried out largely with the use of specific point mutations in bacteria provided compelling evidence for the over-all validity of the code as worked out by Nirenberg and others. The code was found to apply equally to bacteria, plants, and animals and was thus universal.

These brilliant series of studies from Mendel to the breaking of the genetic code have provided evidence of how a gene functions to specify a specific trait. They represent one of the truly great intellectual and experimental achievements in the human endeavor.

The available experimental evidence suggests that, with very few exceptions, all cells of an organism contain a complete complement of genes. This is evidenced by the fact that all of the different specialized cells found in any given species of animal or plant contain the same amount of DNA while the sex cells contain one-half that amount, a finding that was made by Alfred E. Mirsky, whose memory we are honoring in this lecture series, together with his associate Hans Ris (42) as well as by the Vendrelys (43) in England. This is evidenced further by the finding that the progeny of single specialized cells of plants such as tobacco (44) or carrot (45) when isolated and grown under appropriate conditions in culture are capable of developing into completely normal, fully fertile plants. Similarly, when nuclei are isolated from differentiated intestinal epithelial cells of feeding tadpoles of the African clawed toad and implanted into normal toad eggs from which the nucleus has been removed such differentiated nuclei are capable of directing the development of fully mature African clawed toads that are normal in every respect (46). The results of these and other similar studies indicate then that all of the genetic information required to reconstitute an entirely normal organism is retained in the nuclei of cells that have become specialized. If it is true, as the evidence suggests, that all of the different specialized cell types such as liver, kidney, nerve, muscle, skin, etc., that are found in higher animals contain the same complement of genes and if genes code for the specialized properties that are shown by the different specialized cell types, then how does one explain the striking differences that are found to exist between the different types of cells? The answer to that question is simply that only a relatively small number of the total number of genes present in a cell are functional. It is now believed that more than 90 percent of all of the genetic information present in a cell is repressed and hence is nonfunctional. Of the remaining 10 percent of the genes that are active a certain number, such as, for example, those coding for the respiratory enzymes, are functional in all cells since all living cells respire, while those genes that give cells their specialized characteristics are selectively activated or repressed, different ones for the different specialized cell types. Genes required for the production of hemoglobin, the red-colored protein found in red blood cells, are turned on in nucleated red blood cells but not in other cell types, while the genes required to code for another protein, serum albumin, are turned on specifically in liver cells but not in other cell types. With a model such as this it is easy to understand why different cell types found in an organism, although containing the same complement of genes, may be very different in appearance and in the functions that they perform. That this is, in fact, what is happening in a cell can be illustrated very dramatically with the use of giant chromosomes that are found in the salivary glands of certain insects such as, for example, the common fruit fly, _Drosophila_, or the midge, _Chironomus_. These giant chromosomes are much larger than those found in other cells and hence their fine structure is more easily observable. When such chromosomes are stained with appropriate dyes they show many alternating light and dark cross bands (see Fig. 3). Although large, thread-like structures, which we now know were the giant chromosomes, had been observed in cells of the salivary glands of certain insect larvae as early as 1881, it was not until 1933 that they were identified as being chromosomes. In that year Theophilus Painter in this country

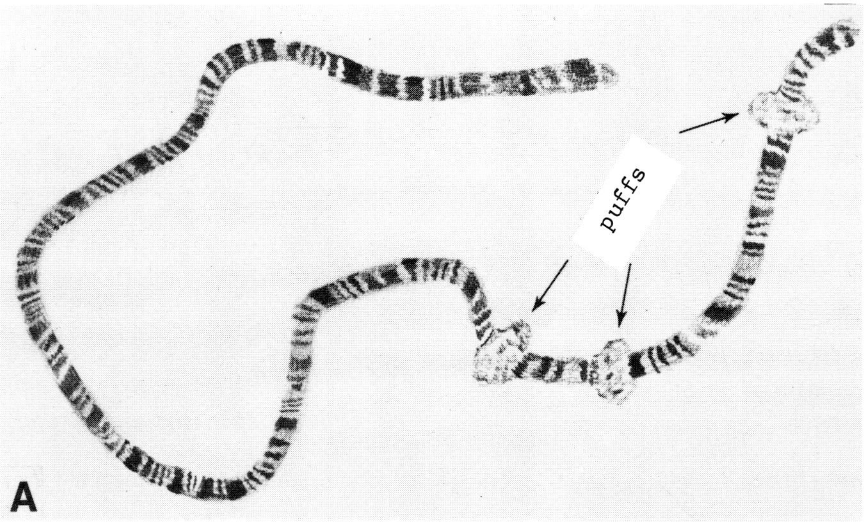


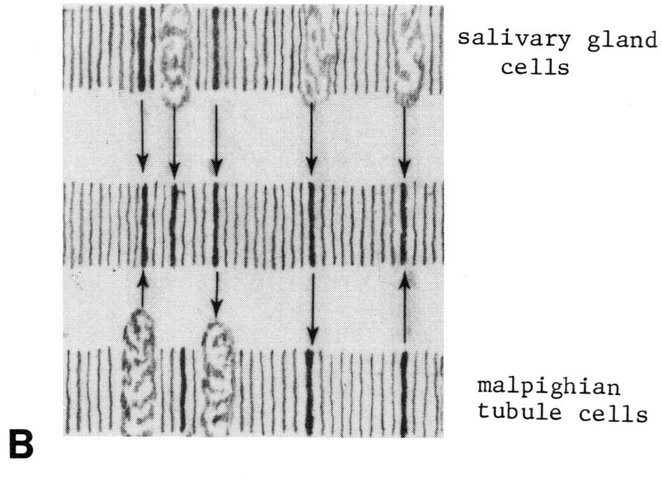


FIGURE 3. (A) A diagrammatic representation of a giant salivary gland chromosome showing light and dark cross bands as well as puffed regions. The puffs represent foci of active RNA synthesis. (B) A diagrammatic sketch of the same segment of a giant chromosome found in salivary gland cells and in malpighian tubule cells showing that different bands are puffed in the same chromosome segment of the two cell types.

showed that the cross bands observed on the giant chromosomes correspond to specific gene loci as determined by genetic studies (47, 48). An analysis by C.B. Bridges in 1935 of the four chromosomes that are present in salivary gland cells of *Drosophila* showed that one of these, the X chromosome, had 725 bands, the second had 1320 bands, the third 1450 bands, while a fourth small chromosome had 45 recognizable cross bands (49). The suggestion that the bands correspond to gene loci received experimental support from the studies of W. Beermann and his associates in Germany, as well as others working elsewhere, who found that although the banding patterns were identical in the same chromosome found in different specialized cell types of the organism, the individual bands found on the chromosomes showed characteristic differences in appearance in the different cell types. Particular bands, different ones for different cell types, were swollen into puffs (see Fig. 3). These puffed regions were found, moreover, to be centers of active RNA synthesis. Beermann presented conclusive evidence that a puff represented an active gene locus by correlating the presence of a specific puffed region in a chromosome of a specific cell type in the midge *Chironomus* with the ability of that cell type to produce specific proteinaceous granules. That same band was in a condensed or nonpuffed form in the same cell type found in an insect that did not produce the specific granules. A detailed analysis showed that the specific genetic locus responsible for the synthesis of these proteinaceous granules was located at the distal end of chromosome 4 in _Chironomus_. A correlation was found to exist, moreover, between the presence of a puff at the specific gene locus in special salivary gland cells of _Chironomus pallidivittatus_ and an ability to synthesize granules while no puff was observed at that same gene locus in the closely related _Chironomus tentans_ species which did not synthesize the proteinaceous granules. When these two insect species were hybridized and the progeny of the cross studied a perfect correlation was again found to exist between the presence of a puff at the specific gene locus and an ability to synthesize the particular proteinaceous product (50). It has been found, moreover, that somewhere around 10 percent of the gene loci on any given chromosome are in a puffed or active form while the rest are in the condensed or inactive form. These studies provide excellent visible evidence then for the concept of active and inactive gene states within cells and account for the fact that although very different kinds of cells of a given species of plant or animal contain the same complement of genes, those cells are different, one from another, because different genes are functional in the different kinds of cells.

The question that arises next, therefore, is what are the factors and regulatory mechanisms that determine which of the genes in a cell are active and which are repressed. It has been found, for example, that the characteristic puff patterns can be modified by specific environmental factors. It is known that the insect hormone ecdysone induces molting in an insect. If this hormone is administered before pupation would normally occur the puff pattern found on the chromosomes changes rapidly to that characteristic of the pupation stage and molting then takes place. Other hormones have now been found to selectively activate genes experimentally in test systems other than those involving insects. A striking example of this is found in the case of the effects of the female sex hormone estrogen on the synthesis of two special proteins by the chicken. It is well known that when an egg is being formed in a hen the estrogen produced by the hen's ovaries stimulates its liver to produce two egg yolk proteins which are known as phosvitin and lipovitellin. These proteins are not normally produced by a rooster. However, if estrogen is administered to a rooster its liver will now produce very significant amounts of these two egg yolk proteins. It would be difficult indeed to find a more dramatic instance of the selective activation by a specific substance of normally repressed genes than is provided by the example cited above.

There are, in addition, the as yet largely uncharacterized cytoplasmic factors and mechanisms that play a central role in regulating nuclear gene expression during the normal course of development of an organism. We have already noted the profound effects that the egg cytoplasm exerts on the developmental potentialities of nuclei obtained from differentiated intestinal epithelial cells of the African clawed toad. The results of that study demonstrate that the differentiated nucleus not only retains all of the genetic information necessary to reconstitute an entirely normal toad but that the genetic information present in that nucleus can be reprogramed in such a way by the egg cell cytoplasm that the progeny of that nucleus give rise to all of the specialized cell types found in an adult toad. Many of the early embryological studies, particularly those dealing with the development in amphibians such as newts and frogs, pointed to the importance of the cytoplasm in influencing nuclear gene activity. The essential structure of an amphibian egg at the time of fertilization is quite simple. Yolk platelets tend to concentrate at the lower or vegetal pole of the egg while the nucleus is commonly found at the upper or animal pole. Soon after fertilization of the egg a further regional difference appears. A special cytoplasmic region known as the gray crescent is found slightly below the equator of the egg cell and is concentrated toward the main axis of the egg (see Fig. 4). This special cytoplasmic region plays an extremely important role in the early development of the organism. This is evidenced by the fact that if, for example, a newt egg is pinched in two in such a way that the nucleus and gray crescent are present in one of the halves, that half of the egg will develop into a normal adult newt. If, on the other hand, one half of an egg that contains a nucleus but not the gray crescent material is allowed to develop, the cells will grow and divide but they will not produce any of the characteristic features of adult tissues. Such cells remain embryonic and without a capacity for specific differentiation. It is clear, therefore, that the gray crescent material present in the cytoplasm plays a most important role in programing nuclear gene function during the early development of the organism.

Other very important cellular mechanisms that regulate metabolic activity in a cell are the membranes which surround not only the cell itself but organelles such as the mitochondria and the nucleus that are present in cells. These membranes represent semipermeable barriers that very largely determine what gets into and out of a cell and its organelles from the immediate environment and in this way play a most important role in regulating cellular metabolism.

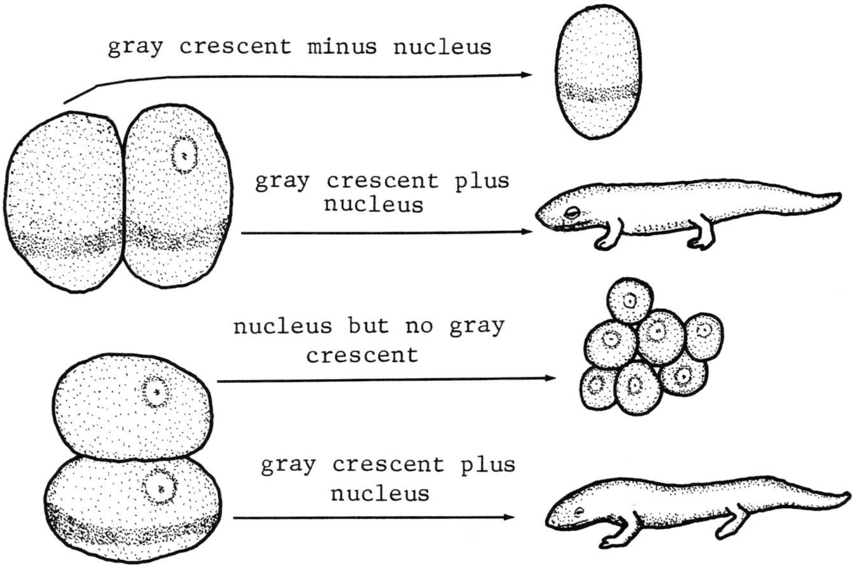


FIGURE 4. Experiments of the type pictured above illustrate the importance of the cytoplasm of a cell in directing early development and cellular differentiation. Activated eggs of certain vertebrates such as the newt contain a readily recognizable cytoplasmic region that is known as the gray crescent. If a newt egg is pinched in two in such a way that one cell contains both a nucleus and gray crescent-containing cytoplasm that cell will produce an adult, fully functional newt. If a cell contains gray crescent material but no nucleus, that cell will not develop further. If, on the other hand, an egg is pinched in two in such a way that one of the eggs contains a nucleus but no gray crescent-containing cytoplasm the cell may undergo division but the resulting cells never produce any of the characteristic features found in adult tissues. The cells remain embryonic without a capacity for specific differentiation. Only if both a nucleus and gray crescent material are present will normal development proceed. It is thus the gray crescent material found in the cytoplasm that first switches on nuclear gene activities that control the synthesis of proteins concerned with cellular differentiation.

There are other much better defined types of regulatory mechanisms that control the action of genes in cells. These have been most thoroughly studied in organisms such as the bacteria. There are, for example, enzymes--the so-called inducible enzymes--which are produced by cells only in response to the presence of the specific molecules on which those enzymes act. Using such a system two French scientists, François Jacob and Jacques Monod, together with their associates brilliantly worked out and described such a system of gene regulation in the bacteria (51). In this particular instance the regulatory system consists of four units: (1) a regulatory gene, (2) an operator, (3) a structural gene, and (4) a permease structural gene which allows a specific substance (in this instance, β galactoside which induces the formation of a specific enzyme, β galactosidase) to penetrate the bacterial cell. In the absence of the specific substance, a repressor present in the cell interacts with the operator in such a way that the information present in the DNA of the structural gene is not transcribed into its mRNA equivalent. Thus the specific enzyme β galactosidase is not produced. If, on the other hand, the substrate (β galactoside) is present it combines with the repressor molecule and inactivates it. The operator then becomes functional and the enzymes necessary to utilize the substrate β galactoside are produced. Thus, whether the specific gene is turned on or off is determined, in this instance, by whether a specific substrate is present or absent in a cell. While such a system of gene regulation doubtless applies to organisms such as the bacteria and other lower forms, the regulatory systems are perhaps more complicated and certainly far less well understood in cells of higher organisms.

There are, in addition, numerous types of regulatory mechanisms found in a cell which operate below the level of the gene. One of the best understood of this type of regulatory mechanism is known as feedback inhibition which involves the specific inhibition--not the formation--of one of the enzymes which often is at or near the beginning of a sequence of reactions in a multienzyme system. An enzyme in this sequence, which is inhibited by the end product of the reaction, is known as an allosteric enzyme because it not only contains a specific site for binding its substrate, as do all enzymes, but it also contains a specific site for binding a modulator which it does not catalyze but which inhibits its catalytic activity for its specific substrate. Thus, as shown in Figure 5, tryptophan, which is the end product of the reaction chain that leads in four steps to the synthesis of that amino acid, inhibits the enzyme that converts chorismic acid to anthranilic acid and thus regulates the level of

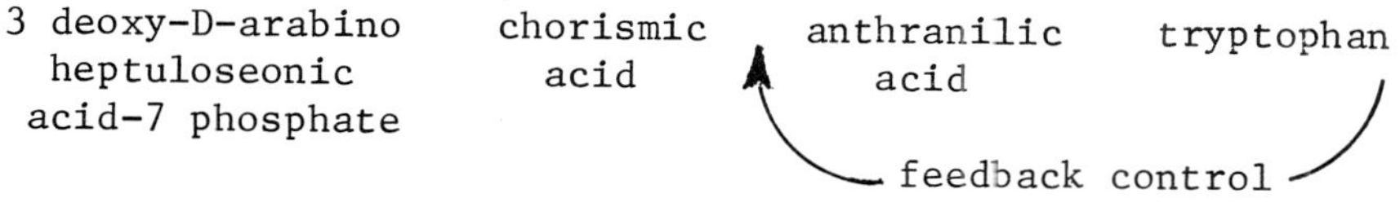


FIGURE 5. A type of regulatory mechanism, known as feedback inhibition, which operates below the level of the gene. Control mechanisms of this type involve the inhibition--not the formation--of one of the enzymes in a multienzyme system by the end product (tryptophan) of the reaction. In this particular instance tryptophan inhibits an enzyme that is involved in the conversion of chorismic acid to anthranilic acid and thus regulates the level of tryptophan in a cell.

tryptophan produced in a cell. Allosteric enzymes may thus serve an important regulatory role in cellular metabolism. Other types of regulatory enzymes are the so-called covalently modulated enzymes which are interconvertible between active and inactive states by the action of other enzymes. The isozymes, which occur as multiple forms of the same enzyme, within a given species or cell type represent another form of regulatory enzymes. Although different isozymes of the same enzyme catalyze the same basic reaction, not only the rates of reaction but also the end products of the reaction may differ depending on which of the isozymes predominates in a cell.

These are but some of the regulatory mechanisms that control metabolism and an understanding of those mechanisms is, as we shall see later, essential for an understanding of the cancer problem.

These, then, are the major pieces of information that we have available in our attempt to solve the jigsaw puzzle that we know as cancer. If all of the required pieces have now been identified we need only to fit them into their proper places to gain an understanding of the nature of that disease. If, on the other hand, some few pieces of the puzzle are still unaccounted for it may, nevertheless, be possible for us to see the broad outline of the picture that our puzzle is designed to depict. If major parts of the puzzle are still missing, then we will, of course, be unsuccessful in our efforts. Our problem now will be to attempt to arrange the available pieces as skillfully as possible to learn whether we can arrive at a reasonable understanding of that ghastly enigma that is known to us as cancer.

# CHAPTER II

# DISTINGUISHING CHARACTERISTICS OF TUMOR CELLS

In setting out to analyze a problem as complex as the tumor problem it would first appear necessary to clearly define the distinguishing characteristics of tumor cells in general and of malignant or cancer cells in particular. True tumor cells, which are also known as neoplastic (meaning new growth) cells, have been divided into two broad categories which include the benign tumors, on the one hand, and the malignant tumors or cancers on the other. The distinction between the benign and malignant state is, however, by no means always easy to make even for an experienced pathologist since tumors with intermediate properties exist.

A tumor cell, whether benign or malignant, is a persistently altered cell that reproduces true to type and against the growth of which there is usually no adequate control mechanism in a host. That statement simply means that during the conversion of a normal cell into a tumor cell a profound and heritable change occurs which allows the tumor cell to determine its own activities largely irrespective of the laws that govern so precisely the growth of all normal cells in an organism. This newly acquired property, which is known as autonomy, is the most important single characteristic of tumor cells since without it there would be no tumors.

## BENIGN TUMORS

The benign tumors are characterized by the fact that they commonly remain localized at the site of origin in their host and their growth is often sharply delimited. Benign tumors of many different kinds are found to occur in animals and humans and most of these, such as, for example, a wart or a common dermal nevus of the skin, are quite harmless. However, when benign tumors develop in certain vital tissues and organs they may disrupt function and may even cause death. Some of these benign tumors, such as the ovarian tumors found in human females, may grow to enormous size and tumors weighing 70 pounds or more have been described. Benign tumors of the skin, such as the keratomas which develop in animals, may also reach huge size and may ultimately kill their hosts by simply overwhelming them (see Fig. 6).

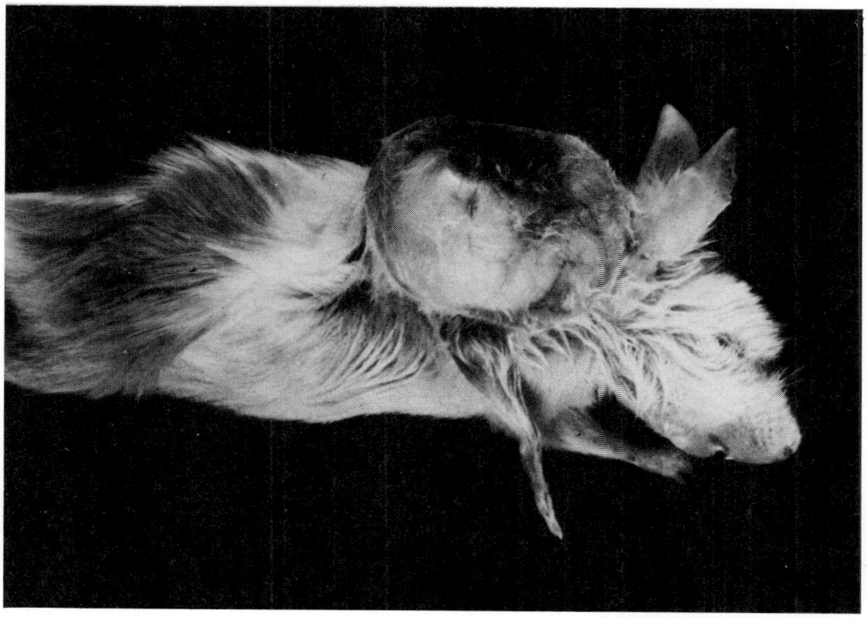

FIGURE 6. A benign and transplantable tumor (keratoma) of the mouse that does not commonly invade or metastasize but ultimately overwhelms and kills its host as a result of continued growth. This type of tumor may occasionally give rise to cells that invade and metastasize and thus becomes malignant in the clinical sense. The capacities to invade and metastasize may therefore be secondarily acquired characteristics and may be dismissed in any consideration of the earliest event responsible for the conversion of a normal cell to a tumor cell which is the development by a tumor cell of a capacity for autonomous growth. (Courtesy of Dr. James S. Henderson)

Cells of benign tumors retain many of the characteristic features of the normal cells from which they are derived. They are, therefore, classified by pathologists according to the specific cell types from which they arise. Thus, if benign tumors arise from skin cells they are known as papillomas, keratomas, pigmented moles, warts, etc., depending on the type of skin cell from which they are derived. If they arise from connective tissue cells they are known as fibromas, from fat cells as lipomas, from immature nerve cells as ganglioneuromas, from bone as osteomas, from muscle as myomas, from glands as adenomas, etc.

## MALIGNANT TUMORS

Malignant tumors, unlike benign tumors, do not remain localized in their hosts during later stages of their development and their growth is often diffuse rather than being sharply delimited. Such tumors are characterized by the fact that they invade and destroy surrounding normal tissues and detach small groups of cells which then move or metastasize through the blood vessels or lymph channels to distant sites in a host where new tumors of the same kind may arise. It is this ability of malignant cells to become widely disseminated in their hosts that makes cancer such a dangerous and often incurable disease.

The malignant tumors have been classified by pathologists into two broad categories, the carcinomas and the sarcomas. The carcinomas are cancers that are derived from epithelial cells, that is, the cells that line the outer and inner surfaces of the body and their derivatives such as those found in the skin, the nose, mouth, throat, stomach, intestines, as well as ducts, glands, nerves, breasts, urinary and genital systems, and organs such as the lungs, kidney, and liver. The sarcomas, on the other hand, arise from the mesenchyme, that is, from cells found in connective tissues and in the supportive tissues such as bone, cartilage, tendons, muscle, and the lymphatics. The malignant tumors, like the benign tumors, are classified by pathologists according to the specific cell types from which they originate. Thus, if cancers are derived from stem cells that give rise to the stratified layer of the skin they are known as squamous cell carcinomas, those arising from pigment cells are named melanomas, those from immature nerve cells neuroblastomas, those from glands adenocarcinomas, while those derived from organs such as, for example, the liver are known as hepatocarcinomas or more commonly as hepatomas. The sarcomas that arise from connective tissue cells are classified as fibrosarcomas, those from muscle as myosarcomas or rhabdomyosarcomas, from bone osteogenic sarcomas, while those that arise from cartilage are known as chondrosarcomas.

Although there is essentially fivefold more connective tissue in humans than there is epithelial tissue, carcinomas are responsible for about 85 percent of all cancers in adults while the sarcomas account for only about 2 percent. It has been found, moreover, that while the rate of the development of sarcomas remains essentially constant at all age levels, carcinomas increase with increasing age (see Fig. 7). The increased incidence of carcinomas with age is generally attributed to the fact that the epithelial cells that line

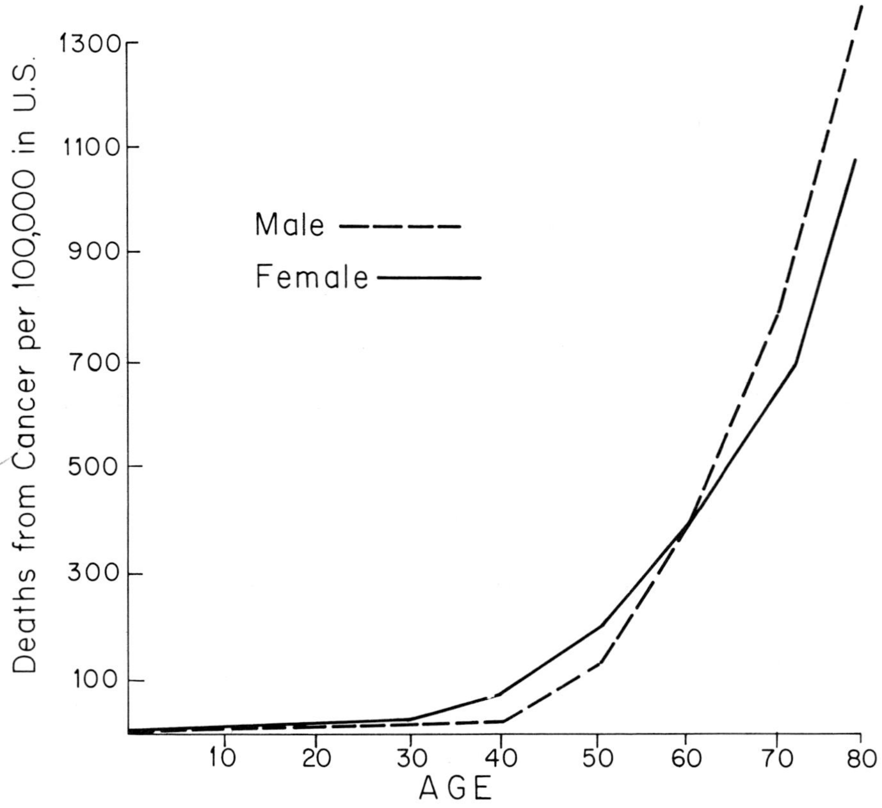


FIGURE 7. Graph showing the relationship of deaths resulting from cancer to age in the United States in 1945.

the outer and inner body surfaces are more directly exposed to and are thus more subject to the cumulative effects of the cancer-producing agents that are ever present in the environment around us.

In addition to the carcinomas and sarcomas there are tumors that originate from the immature white or red blood cells that are known as leukemias. There are certain white blood cells, the granulocytes, that originate in the bone marrow and when such cells become tumorous either a chronic or an acute myelocytic leukemia results. In either case, there is an enormous increase in the number of leukemic granulocytes in the peripheral blood. Sometimes, however, the leukemic cells do not enter the blood stream but pile up where they are produced and displace the normal blood-forming bone marrow with tumor marrow. When a second type of white blood cell, the lymphocytes, which arise in the lymphatic tissues, becomes cancerous the resulting diseases are known as lymphocytic leukemia. Here again, the form of the disease may be either chronic or acute and in either case there is found an enormous increase in leukemic lymphocytes in the blood. If the cancerous lymphocytes multiply but remain localized they give rise to solid tumor masses and then are known as lymphomas or lymphosarcomas. When immature red blood cells become neoplastic the resulting condition is known as erythroid leukemia. The leukemias account for 3.4 percent while the lymphomas account for 5.4 percent of the diagnosed malignancies. The remaining approximately 5 percent of tumors are not readily classifiable and are derived from mixed tissues such as those found in testes and ovaries.

Since cells of each tissue present in the body can give rise to a whole spectrum of benign and malignant tumors, the classification presented above is, of course, quite incomplete and is intended only to give the reader some idea of the nomenclature used by the tumor pathologist to classify tumors. Many of the tumors identified above will be referred to again during the course of this discussion. The classification of tumors is done not merely to satisfy curiosity but such a classification is of great practical value to the medical profession. It has been found through long experience that the structure and appearance of a tumor and the cells of which it is composed are closely associated with its activities in a host. Thus, a pathologist when examining a tumor with a microscope can often give invaluable advice concerning a prognosis as well as the probable sensitivity of particular tumors to therapy.

## CHARACTERISTIC FEATURES OF TUMOR CELLS

### A. Autonomy

The tumorous state thus clearly manifests itself in many different ways. Some tumors grow very slowly in their hosts while others grow very rapidly. It should be noted, however, that even some of the most rapidly growing tumors do not grow at a faster rate than do some normal cell types. When, for example, three-fourths of the normal liver of an animal or man is removed the remaining liver cells will regenerate the complete organ in two to three weeks time. Tumors of the liver seldom if ever achieve comparable growth rates. Growth of the normal regenerating liver cells is, moreover, precisely regulated and when the organ has been reconstituted, growth of the normal liver cells promptly stops. Growth of liver tumors is, of course, essentially unrestrained and, if malignant, will destroy that organ. It is not, therefore, merely rapid growth that is important to the tumor problem but rather the development by tumor cells of a capacity for unrestrained or autonomous growth. Some tumors, as has been indicated, remain localized at the site of their origin while others invade and destroy surrounding normal tissues and become widely disseminated in their hosts. Tumors that remain localized may, during later periods of their growth, give rise to cells that invade and metastasize and thus become malignant in the clinical sense. That this can and does occur indicates that the capacities to invade and metastasize may be acquired, sometimes relatively late, and may therefore be dismissed in a search for the earliest event responsible for the heritable cellular change that underlies the tumorous state. Some tumors have been found to invade underlying normal tissues extensively but to rarely metastasize, while certain other tumors become widely disseminated in their hosts despite a minimum capacity to invade and destroy normal tissues. Thus an ability to invade, to metastasize, or simply to grow autonomously are dissociable characters that may be inherited independently of one another (52). Explanations as to why tumor cells grow autonomously and why they may invade and metastasize represent very important pieces in our cancer puzzle and an attempt will be made to provide insight into those problems later in this discussion.

The cells of many tumors retain, as has been indicated, certain of the specialized functions that characterize the normal cell type from which they originated. Some of the more slowly growing but malignant and transplantable Morris hepatomas, for example, deviate minimally from normal liver cells both in their structure and function. Other tumors, as we shall see later, acquire specialized functions that are not characteristic of the cell type from which they were derived but rather those of certain other cell types. Cells of some cancers, on the other hand, show such a pronounced deterioration of form and function that it is often very difficult if not impossible for even an experienced pathologist to determine the cell type from which the cancer was derived. The loss of structure and function by cells of certain cancers often results from a dedifferentiation (loss of specialized function) of those cells. Such poorly differentiated tumors are referred to as being anaplastic. It is clear, therefore, that the tumorous state can express itself in many different ways. All true tumor cells have, nevertheless, one thing in common and that is they have acquired a capacity to grow in an essentially unrestrained or autonomous fashion in their hosts.

B. Transplantability

A second characteristic of many true tumor cells, whether they are classified as benign or malignant, is that of transplantability. When small fragments of tumor tissue about the size of the tip of a match are implanted under the skin of appropriate animals, the living tumor cells will grow and develop into new tumors of the same kind from which the implanted cells were derived. Whether grafts of this kind are successful is determined by a number of host-related factors. Although there have been occasional reports of successful tumor grafts between different but closely related animal species such as, for example, the rabbit and the hare, success is generally achieved only when grafts are made to animals belonging to the same species from which the tumor was derived. Even when tumor cells are implanted into members of the same species the number of successful takes may be small during the first passage. The number of successful grafts may be increased very significantly when cells of tumors that develop in a highly inbred line of animals, all members of which are genetically the same, are implanted into other members of that inbred line. Tumor cells may thus be subject to the same host-protective measures as are normal cells since it is well known that normal skin grafts are most successful if skin used for the graft is obtained from the same individual on whom the graft is made or from an identical twin if by chance one is available, while skin from others, even related individuals, is often rejected by the host.

There are certain privileged places in an animal where the host-protective factors responsible for rejection of cells are not functional. One of these is the anterior chamber of the eye and it is possible to successfully grow tumor tissues from very different species in such places. Even cancers from human patients may be successfully grown in anterior chambers of the eyes of rabbits. With the availability of so-called nude mice, which lack a thymus gland and hence a significant part of the normal immune system, many tumors that originate in other animal species including cancers of human origin can also be successfully grown. The cheek pouch of the hamster is another privileged sanctuary where tumor cells of foreign origin can readily be grown.

Cells of many different cancers such as, for example, the Jensen rat sarcoma, Ehrlich's mouse carcinoma, and the Rous VX carcinomas of the rabbit, as well as benign tumors such as a mouse keratoma have been transplanted serially in their respective hosts and have largely retained for many years the characteristic features of the tumor from which they were derived. Since these tumors retain through many transplant generations their characteristic properties, the transplantation studies show that a profound and heritable change has occurred that allows a tumor cell to determine its own activities largely irrespective of the laws that govern so precisely the growth of all normal cells in an organism. A characterization of the precise nature of that heritable cellular change represents another of the main pieces of our cancer puzzle and will be the subject of further analysis later in this discussion.

### C. Oncogenesis as a Multistep Process

The conversion of a normal cell into a rapidly growing, fully autonomous tumor cell may occur either in a single step or as a multistep process, progressing by a series of continuous (gradual) or discontinuous (abrupt) changes from an incipient tumor cell to the fully malignant state. Certain cancer-producing chemicals when applied to the skin of experimental animals in subthreshold amounts may convert normal cells into tumor cells which do not develop into tumorous growths. Such latent tumor cells require a second substance such as croton oil, which is not in itself cancer-producing, to stimulate the latent tumor cells into active growth (53-55). Stimulating substances such as croton oil are known as promoters or cocarcinogens. Thus, tumor formation may be divided into two steps which have come to be known as initiation and promotion. Progression to ever greater malignancy may require additional steps and each step in such a multistage process may be facilitated by specific chemicals that may not be active as promoters in the earlier stages. When tumors proceed through a series of steps from the benign to the malignant state or from the malignant to a more malignant state the phenomenon is known as tumor progression.

It should perhaps be pointed out here that by no means all cancer cells present in an individual develop into overt cancers. There is an abundance of evidence to show that cancer cells, although present, may exist in a latent or silent form, often for years without growing into detectable tumors. It is a not uncommon experience among clinicians to find tumors of the same type arising at different locations often many years after a primary cancer had apparently been successfully removed surgically. This is evidenced further by the finding that routine examinations of "normal" thyroids in older people in one study disclosed that half contained one or more nodules and of these almost half showed histological evidence that was suggestive of thyroid cancers. Yet such a number is very much higher than is the death rate of thyroid cancer which is estimated to be six per million. Thus the protective forces present in a host may keep many cancer cells in check.

## D. Conditional Tumors

Finally, it should be noted that how a tumor develops in its host may be determined by the environment in which the tumor is growing. This point is particularly well illustrated in the so-called conditional or hormone-dependent tumors of animals and plants. Conditional prostate or breast tumors of mammals, which may be highly malignant, may grow only so long as the appropriate hormonal stimulus is present. When the specific stimulus is withdrawn growth of such tumors stops and they may regress, but when the hormonal stimulus is restored growth of the remaining tumor cells begins again. Since these conditional tumors are particularly vulnerable to hormonal manipulation in their host, a strategy based on depriving such tumors of the specific hormone that they require for growth has been widely used as a therapeutic measure. Conditional tumors may undergo progression to a hormone-independent state during their development in a host and then they become true tumors that no longer depend on the specific hormonal stimulus for their continued growth.

### E. Effects of Tumors on Their Hosts

These, then, are the essential characteristics of tumor cells in general and malignant cells in particular. What, then, briefly, are the effects of such cells on the hosts in which they develop? Although many of the debilitating effects that cancers have on their hosts are as yet poorly understood it is clear that different types of cancer affect their hosts in different ways. Some do this by seriously disrupting essential functions of vital organs while others such as those of the endocrine (hormone secreting) glands continue to produce large amounts of their specific hormones even when still very small in size. Such cancers may be highly toxic and even lethal due to the excessive production of their specific hormones. Still others may cause respiratory failure or cardiovascular insufficiency. All tumors are characterized by the fact that they grow at the expense of their hosts. They behave as parasites and they may thrive despite relative starvation of the hosts in which they develop. This may be illustrated in the case of lipomas or fat tumors but is true of many other tumors as well. In a well nourished individual the reserve material is stored as fat. Such reserve fat is readily consumed by the body when the need arises. Lipomas contain fat that is chemically the same as that normally deposited in the body and yet the lipoma does not shrink in size even though the reserve fat present in a host in which such lipomas develop is completely utilized as the result of a wasting disease or other cause. Tumors thus have a priority on the body's economy and have a tendency to continue to grow even when the rest of the body suffers from relative starvation. It is this ability to live at the expense of their host, particularly in the case of widely disseminated tumors, that leads to extreme loss of weight and typical debilitation known as "cachexia" that is so characteristic of patients with advanced cancer. Such patients are often so weakened that they die not from the cancer but from secondary infections mostly bacterial in nature.

Cancers have, moreover, an ability to manipulate the activity and behavior of the normal tissues of their hosts in such a way as to ensure the survival of the cancer at the expense of and to the detriment of the host. Many tumors have a so-called "stroma" which is commonly composed of a network of connective tissue. There are blood vessels present in the stroma that supply the tumor with oxygen and nutrients and remove metabolic wastes from the tumor. Without these blood vessels the malignant cells could not survive, at least not in large masses. It has been found that the cancer cells themselves produce a specific substance, known as the tumor angiogenesis factor, which acts to specifically induce the formation of the new blood vessels (see Fig. 28, Chapter 8). Thus, by cleverly, almost diabolically, manipulating the cells of the host the cancer ensures not only its survival but provides an environment suitable for its continued well being all at the expense of the host.

Cancer is a disease of stealth and the relationship

between cancers and their hosts is often so insidious that the malignant cells become widely disseminated in their hosts before a diagnosis of the disease is made. It is this fact that makes cancer so difficult to cope with and makes it such a dangerous and often incurable disease.

# CHAPTER III

## THE DEVELOPMENT OF AUTONOMY

Tumor cells have often been compared to anarchists in an otherwise very beautifully organized and regulated society of cells. While some of the most malignant of the cancers can perhaps quite legitimately be compared to the more violent of the nihilists found in modern societies, other kinds of tumors are not as disruptive and some of the more benign of these are only marginal offenders of the laws. Yet, in all instances, but to different degrees, tumor cells simply do not operate within the prescribed rules that govern so precisely the growth of all normal cells in an organism. In order to understand why the generality of tumor cells behave in an antisocial manner we must first identify the laws that regulate the behavior of all normal cells and then attempt to determine, on the one hand, how those laws are enforced in our society of cells and, on the other, why they are violated by the tumor cells.

## SUBSTANCES AND MECHANISMS THAT REGULATE CELL GROWTH AND DIVISION

Since all tumor cells are characterized by the fact that they grow in an essentially unrestrained or autonomous manner in their hosts while the growth of all normal cells is precisely regulated, it would appear that something has gone radically wrong in the tumor cells with those cellular mechanisms that regulate cell growth and division in all normal cell types. We, fortunately, now know something about the factors and cellular mechanisms that regulate cell growth and division. The normal regulatory mechanisms that are operative in controlling cell growth and division can perhaps best be illustrated with the use of a concept based on the so-called cell cycle. When normal cells of either plant or animal origin are stimulated to divide they proceed through a characteristic cell cycle which consists of distinct phases designated as G1, S, G2, M, and D (see Fig. 8). When such cells prepare to divide they begin to produce the necessary enzymes and specific substances that are required to duplicate their genetic material, the chromosomal DNA. This is accomplished during the late G1 phase of the cell cycle. Once a cell has

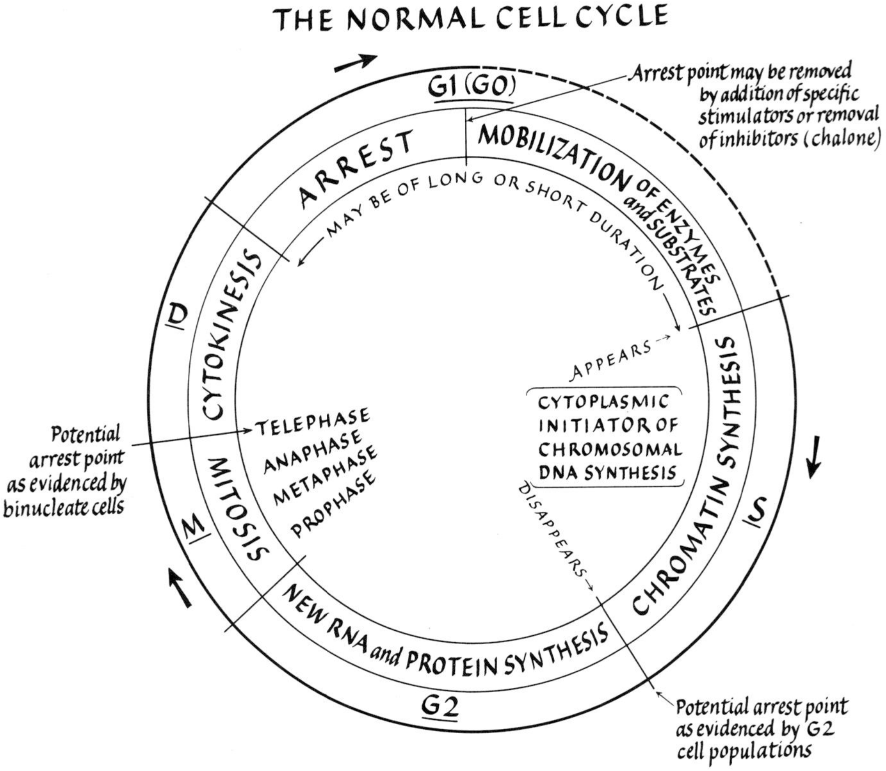


FIGURE 8. Diagram of the normal cell cycle showing different phases of the cycle as well as potential arrest points in the cycle.

produced the required enzymes and precursor substances it begins to synthesize its chromosomal DNA and then enters the S phase of the cell cycle. Chromosomal DNA synthesis is regulated by a cytoplasmic initiator of that process which appears in a cell at the beginning of S phase and disappears again when chromosomal DNA synthesis is complete. Once the genetic material has been duplicated the cell proceeds into the G2 phase of the cell cycle. It is during this phase that new and different enzymes and substrates that are required for nuclear division are produced in a cell. When the nucleus divides the cell is said to be in the M or mitotic phase of the cell cycle. It is also during this phase that the chromosomes containing the genetic information split lengthwise and each member of a divided chromosome is drawn to opposite ends of a cell. In this way a precise distribution of the genetic information present in a cell occurs. Once the chromosomes have aligned themselves at opposite ends of a cell, new nuclei are reconstituted and the cell itself divides by a process known as cytokinesis. This represents the D or division phase of the cell cycle. It is clear that there must be points in the cell cycle in which the cycle is arrested, otherwise the normal cells would continue to proliferate continuously and they would, in effect, behave as do tumor cells. A number of major blocks or arrest points in the cycle have now been identified. The first of these is in the G1 phase of the cell cycle. It is at this point that the normal cell cycle is most commonly arrested. This block can be removed in a resting cell either by the addition of appropriate stimulatory substances or by the removal of tissue-specific inhibitory substances that are known as chalones. A second arrest point in the cycle depends on the absence in a cell of a cytoplasmic initiator of chromosomal DNA synthesis. This cytoplasmic factor can be demonstrated convincingly in a variety of experimental test systems that range from the protozoa (56, 57) to the vertebrates (58, 59) by implanting nuclei in the G1 or G2 phases of the cell cycle into cytoplasm of cells in the S phase of that cycle and showing that these G1- and G2-derived nuclei now actively synthesize chromosomal DNA. Conversely, when S phase nuclei, which are actively synthesizing DNA, are implanted into G1 or G2 phase cytoplasm, DNA synthesis promptly stops. A third major block in the normal cell cycle is found to occur in the G2 phase of the cycle. This block is evidenced by the fact that G2 cell populations are not uncommonly found in higher animal and plant species. These cells can be recognized by the fact that when they are appropriately stimulated they proceed directly into mitosis without again replicating their chromosomal DNA (60). A fourth block that occurs is found between the M and D phases of the cell cycle. This block is evidenced most clearly by the rather common occurrence in both animals and plants of cells in which nuclear division has occurred without corresponding cell division, resulting in cells that contain two or more nuclei. It is these arrest points in the cell cycle that act as the law enforcers that keep growth and division of normal cells in check. It is clear that if blocking mechanisms of this type did not exist, the normal cells would grow and divide persistently in an otherwise suitable environment.

All of the major blocks in the normal cell cycle appear to depend on the absence of one or more specific substances, or at least they can be overcome by specific substances. Even in those instances in which inhibitory substances such as the chalones must be removed from a cell before the cell proceeds through the cell cycle, specific substances must be produced by a cell or provided to a cell if that cell is to proceed through the cell cycle. How, then, are the several arrest points in the cell cycle persistently removed to permit a cell such as a tumor cell to proliferate persistently? In order to gain insight into this question we might profitably turn our attention first to normal and tumor cells of higher plant species. Such systems seem particularly useful for studies of this type because they represent a very complex biological phenomenon in its simplest and most uncomplicated form.

Plant tumors are caused by many of the same general classes of physical, chemical, and biological agents that cause tumors in animals (61). Although, as might be expected, there are some differences in details, tumors found in members of both kingdoms have much in common, as C.O. Jensen first pointed out many years ago. Basic concepts developed with the use of the relatively simple plant tumor systems could therefore well find application and lead to an understanding of the cellular mechanisms that underlie the tumor problem generally.

Insight into the reasons why plant tumor cells proliferate in an unrestrained or autonomous manner in their hosts followed an understanding of the nature of the specific substances that regulate cell growth and division in cells of higher plant species. Growth in all higher animals and plants results either from an enlargement of cells or from the combined processes of cell enlargement and cell division. These fundamental growth processes are controlled in cells of higher plant species by two specific substances, the plant hormone auxin (β-indole-3-acetic acid) and a cell-division-promoting factor. The auxin is concerned with cell enlargement and with chromosomal DNA synthesis while the cell-division-promoting factor acts together with the auxin to promote growth accompanied by cell division. It appears likely that the plant hormone auxin does not initiate chromosomal DNA synthesis directly but rather functions by activating the synthesis in a cell of an as yet uncharacterized substance(s) that is directly involved in that process. The type of experimental approach that permits us to distinguish between these two fundamental growth processes is illustrated in Figure 9. If one isolates specialized cell types such as those found in pith tissue of tobacco or certain other plant species and places those cells on a basic culture medium, the pith cells will not grow. These cells are arrested in the G1 phase of the cell cycle. If, now, one adds a growth substance of the auxin type to the basic medium the individual pith cells enlarge greatly in size and the chromosomal DNA duplicates itself but the cells do not divide. Those cells are blocked in the G2 phase of the cell cycle. Only if a second substance, a cell-division-promoting factor, is added to the culture medium in addition to an auxin will the G2 block be removed and will the treated cells complete the cell cycle. The cell division factor without an auxin is ineffective in promoting either cell enlargement or cell division in the pith cells. Thus, both substances acting in sequence are essential to allow the pith cells to proceed through the cell cycle and complete the division process. It is these two specific substances that remove all of the naturally occurring blocks in the cell cycle. Since precisely the same blocks that arrest the cell cycle in plants exist in cells of animals, it would appear reasonable to assume that those blocks in animal cells are also removed by specific substances. We have seen that in animal cells from the protozoa to the vertebrates

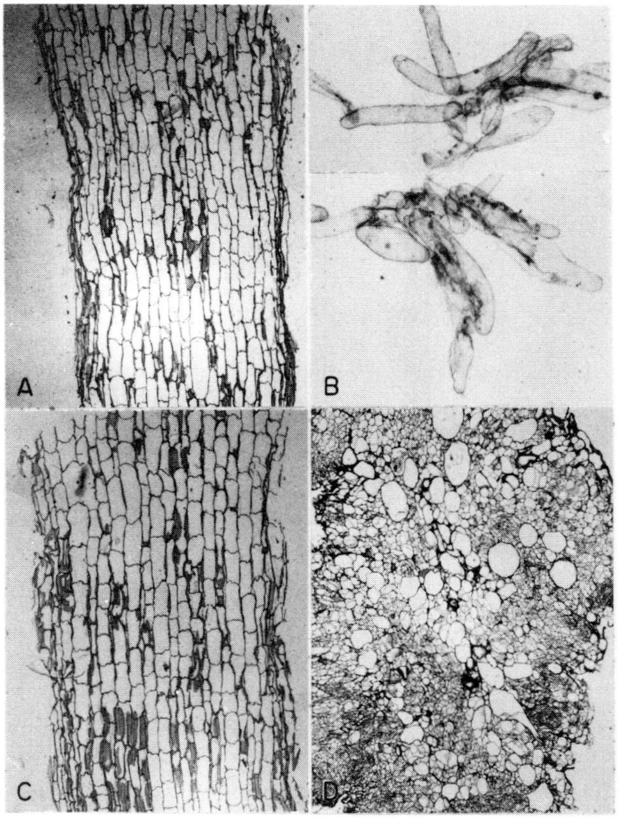


FIGURE 9. The regulation of cell enlargement and cell division in excised pith parenchyma cells of tobacco. Histological sections of (A) control cells planted on a basic culture medium. (B) Basic culture medium supplemented with the plant hormone auxin at a concentration of 1.0 mg/liter of medium. Note the cells have enlarged greatly in size but have not divided. The chromosomal DNA has replicated in cells treated with auxin and they are arrested in the G2 phase of the cell cycle. (C) Basic medium supplemented with a cell-division-promoting factor (6-furfurylaminopurine) at a concentration of 0.5 mg/liter. This compound does not promote cell enlargement, DNA synthesis, or cell division in tobacco pith cells in the absence of auxin. (D) Culture medium supplemented with both an auxin (1.0 mg/liter) and a cell division factor (0.5 mg/liter). Note growth accompanied by cell division results from the synergistic effect of these two growth-regulating substances. (See Fig. 15 B).

a cytoplasmic factor when present in a cell triggers chromosomal DNA synthesis. A protein(s) having a molecular weight of about 50,000 and that is capable of stimulating chromosomal DNA synthesis in isolated nuclei has recently been obtained from extracts of actively proliferating populations of several types of normal cells and from tumor cells but not from similar cells that were in a resting state (62). This appears, therefore, to be the factor that removes the G1 block in the cell cycle in animal cells of mammalian origin. Recent studies have suggested, moreover, that a large molecular weight, nondialyzable substance acts together with the factor that triggers chromosomal DNA synthesis to promote growth accompanied by cell division (63). This nondialyzable component, like the cell division factor in plants, is ineffective in triggering chromosomal DNA synthesis or in promoting cell division in the absence of the factor that encourages DNA synthesis. Thus, although perhaps differing in particulars, the fundamental cellular mechanisms that regulate cell growth and division may be similar in animals and plants.

## DEVELOPMENT OF AUTONOMY IN PLANT TUMOR CELLS

The biosynthetic systems that produce the two essential growth-regulating substances, the auxin and the cell division factor, become repressed and hence nonfunctional when the pith cells become specialized in the developing plant. It was of interest to learn, therefore, how specialized cells would respond if they were converted into tumor cells. The results of studies of this type showed that typical tumors developed when the pith cells were converted into tumor cells (64) (see Fig. 10). What, then, does such a study demonstrate? It shows us that although normal pith cells did not and could not produce either of these two essential growth-regulating substances, following their conversion into tumor cells both of those substances were persistently produced. If that were not true continued growth accompanied by cell division and, hence, tumor formation would not have occurred in that experimental test system. That these two essential growth-regulating substances are, in fact, synthesized persistently by the tumor cells was demonstrated by isolating them from the tumor cells and characterizing them chemically. The continued production of those substances by the tumor cells would appear in itself sufficient to account for the continued abnormal and autonomous growth of those cells.

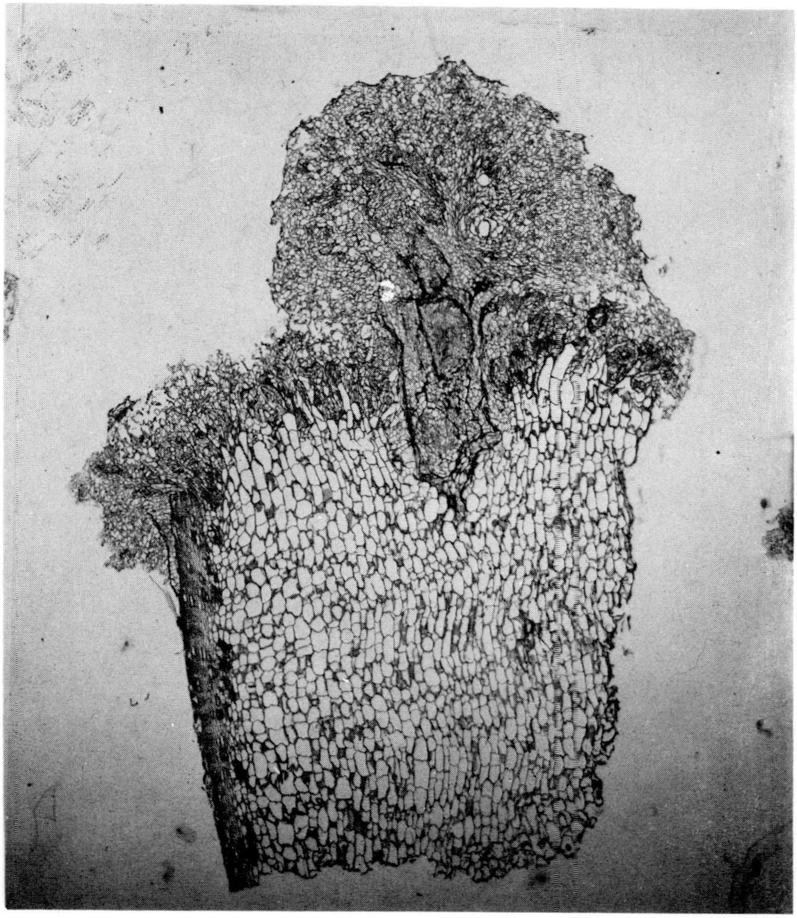

FIGURE 10. Tumor formation in pith parenchyma tissue of tobacco. Although normal tobacco pith cells do not produce either an auxin or a cell-division-promoting factor (see Fig. 9), following the conversion of such cells into tumor cells both of these essential growth-regulating substances are persistently synthesized by the tumor cells. This study demonstrates that a persistent activation of normally repressed biosynthetic systems, the products of which are concerned specifically with cell growth and division, occurs during the transformation of a normal plant cell into a tumor cell.

That this was by no means the entire story was shown by subsequent studies.

It has been found that regardless of cause all true plant tumor cells thus far studied have far simpler growth requirements than do comparable normal cell types. The plant tumor cells proliferate actively and indefinitely on a very simple, chemically defined basic culture medium, composed only of mineral salts, sugar, and three vitamins, that does not support the growth of normal cells of the type from which the tumor cells were derived. This means, of course, that the tumor cells can themselves make all of the essential substances required for their continued growth from the ingredients present in the culture medium. The normal cells, on the other hand, while requiring those substances for growth, cannot make them from the ingredients present in the basic culture medium. What, then, are those essential substances that are manufactured by the tumor cells? In an attempt to find an answer to that question three plant tumor lines derived from the same plant species were used and their growth requirements were compared with those of comparable normal cell types. A comparative study of this type was possible when it was found that the transformation of a normal cell to a rapidly growing, fully autonomous tumor cell does not occur as a single step but takes place progressively over a three- to four-day period. Cells transformed in shorter periods of time grow more slowly in their hosts as well as when they are isolated and planted on a basic culture medium (65) (see Fig. 11). The demonstration of the progressive nature of the crown gall transformation was made possible because of the development of a method that permitted the stopping of the transformation process by means of a thermal treatment at any desired time without affecting the capacity of the host cells that had been transformed prior to the thermal treatment to develop into tumorous growths (66).

The crown gall disease, as was first shown by Erwin F. Smith and C.O. Townsend shortly after the turn of the present century, is caused by a specific bacterium. This bacterium is the cause only in the sense that it very efficiently transmits a tumor-inducing principle which, in turn, is directly responsible for the transformation of normal plant cells into tumor cells (66a). Once the cellular transformation has been accomplished by the tumor-inducing principle the continued abnormal and autonomous proliferation of the transformed cells becomes an automatic process that is entirely independent of the inciting bacteria. In addition to the tumor-inducing principle, it has long been recognized that wounded host tissue is necessary if tumors are to be initiated in the crown gall disease. When a wound is made in the stem

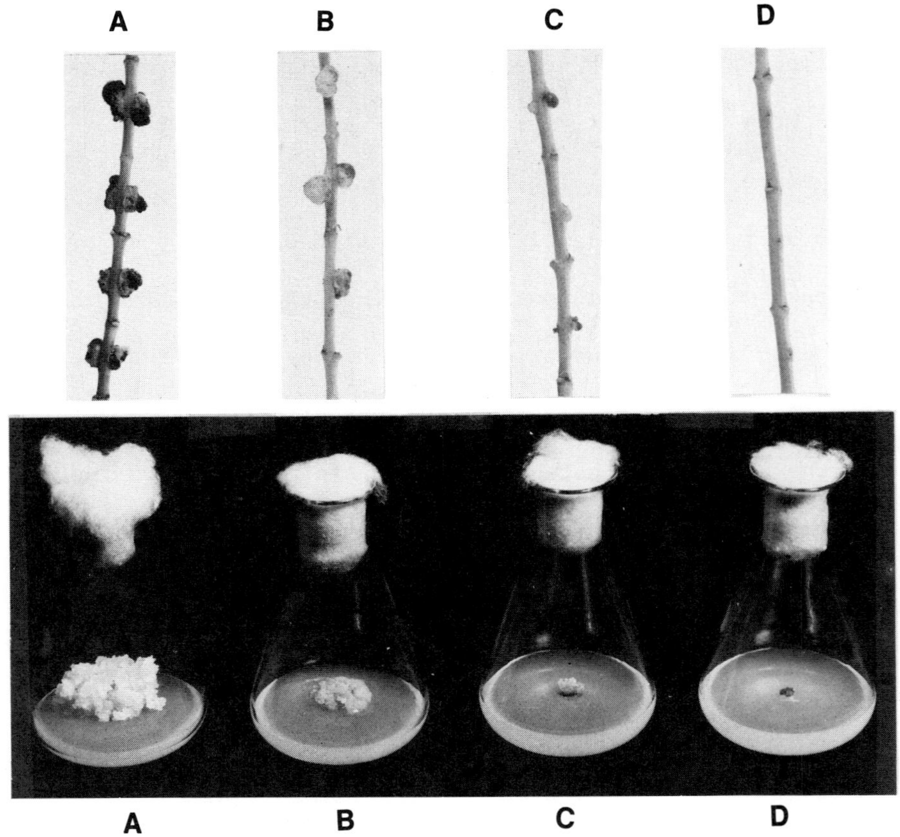


FIGURE 11. Experiment showing the relationship of time that the transformation process was allowed to proceed to the size and rate of growth of the resulting tumors in the crown gall disease of plants. Upper row: Stems of the Madagascar periwinkle inoculated with the transforming bacteria. The bacteria were allowed to act on the plant cells for (A) 72 hours, (B) 60 hours, (C) 34 hours, and (D) control, after which time the bacteria were destroyed by thermal treatment. Lower row shows rate of growth of cells isolated from tumors that developed on stems (A), (B), and (C) and grown on a basic culture medium. Normal control cells (D) did not grow on that culture medium. The three types of tumor cells retained indefinitely in culture their characteristic growth patterns.

of a plant with, say, an ordinary dissecting needle, the cells in the region of the wound are stimulated to divide and within a week to ten days the wound has healed. It has been found that if a susceptible plant species is inoculated with crown gall bacteria and the bacteria are allowed to act on the plant cells for only 24 hours before being killed by thermal treatment no tumors are produced. If the bacteria are allowed to act for 34 to 36 hours before being destroyed, very small, slowly growing tumors result. A 50- to 60-hour exposure of the plant cells to the bacteria results in the development of tumors that grow at a moderately fast rate, while if the bacteria act for 72 to 96 hours before being killed, rapidly growing tumors result (see Figs. 11 and 12). When sterile tumor tissues of the very slowly growing, the moderately fast growing, and very fast growing types are isolated and planted on a basic culture medium they retain indefinitely in culture their characteristic growth patterns.

The fact that a period of somewhat more than 30 hours following inoculation of the plants with the bacteria is required for the first evidence that the cellular transformation has occurred suggests either that that length of time is required for the bacteria to establish themselves in a host and multiply to numbers sufficient to accomplish the cellular transformation, or that a period of somewhat more than 30

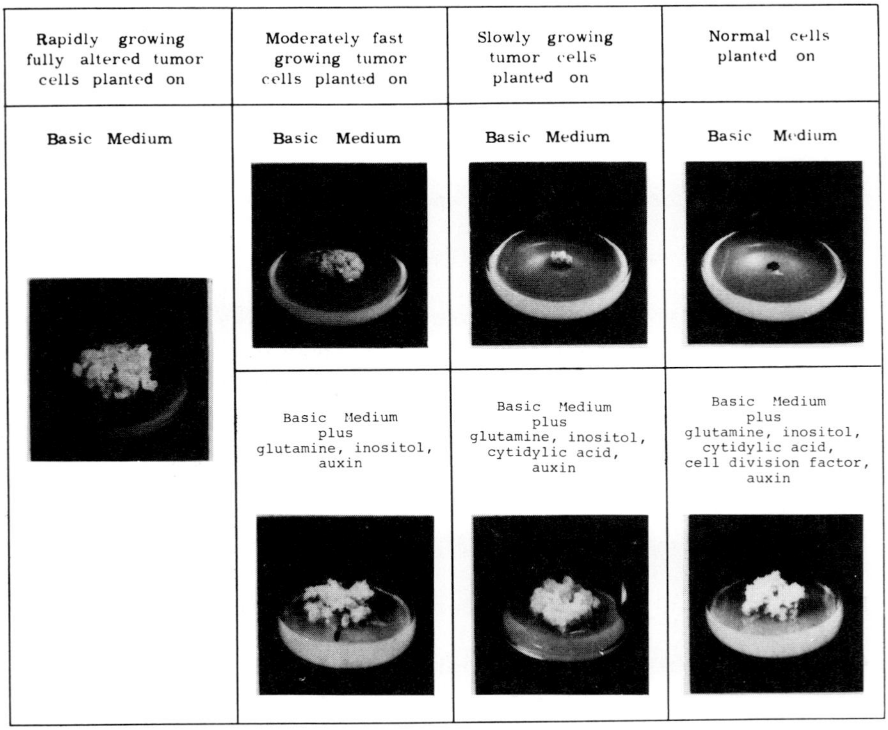


FIGURE 12. Experiment showing the growth-regulating substances and metabolites required to achieve growth rates of normal cells and of the slow growing and moderately fast growing tumor cells equal to that of the fast growing tumor cells grown on a basic culture medium. Cells of the rapidly growing tumor line can make all of the essential growth substances required for their continued rapid growth from the mineral salts, sucrose, and three vitamins present in the basic culture medium. The normal cells cannot do this; they must be supplied with all of the essential growth-promoting substances that the tumor cells make from the ingredients present in the basic culture medium. Cells of the slow and moderately fast growing tumor lines can also synthesize all of the substances needed for their continued growth from the ingredients present in the basic culture medium but not in amounts sufficient for optimal growth.

hours following a wound is required to render the host cells susceptible to transformation. This question was resolved very simply by comparing the response of host cells in the region of a wound that had been allowed to heal for 48 hours prior to inoculation with the bacteria with the response obtained when the bacteria were inoculated directly into previously unwounded tissues. In both instances the bacteria were allowed to act on the host cells for only 24 hours, after which time the transformation process was stopped with a thermal treatment. The results of these experiments are pictured in Figure 13. These studies showed that the host cells became gradually more vulnerable to transformation following a wound, reaching a maximum susceptibility between 48 and 72 hours, after which time they again became more resistant to transformation as wound healing progressed toward completion (67). Thus we see that if the host cells are not competent for transformation, as appears to be the case during the early and late stages of the wound healing process as well as in normal plant cells that are not under the influence of a wound, the cellular transformation will not occur despite the presence of many virulent bacteria in intimate contact with the plant cells. The rendering of cells in the region of a wound competent for transformation is, then, a transient phenomenon and it is only during a less than

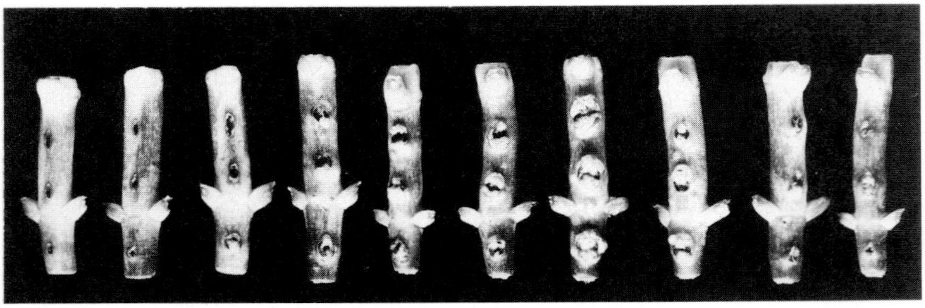

0 3 6 12 18 24 48 72 96 120

Wound healing period in hours prior to transformation

FIGURE 13. Experiments of the type that illustrate the influence of irritation resulting from a wound on the development of competence for cellular transformation in the crown gall disease of plants. Stems of plants shown above were wounded with a sterile needle at three points. The wounded areas were allowed to heal for the period of time in hours indicated above. The transforming bacteria were then introduced into the wounded areas and in all instances allowed to act on the cells in the region of the wound for only 24 hours. Note the host cells become gradually more vulnerable to transformation, reaching a maximum susceptibility when cells in the region of a wound are allowed to heal for 48 hours followed by a 24-hour period of transformation. Thereafter the cells become progressively more resistant to transformation. Thus, if plant cells are not rendered competent as a result of wounding they cannot be transformed into tumor cells despite the presence of many transforming bacteria in intimate contact with those cells.

24-hour period in the total wound healing cycle of 120 hours that normal plant cells can be transformed into tumor cells of the most rapidly growing type. The results of these and other studies show that the effects of the tumor-inducing principle are cumulative up to three to four days, leading in that period of time to fully transformed, rapidly growing tumor cell types (68). There are many instances reported in the animal literature in which the effects of a carcinogen have been found to be cumulative.

Histological studies made of cells during various stages in the wound healing cycle have shown that it is just before the first evidence of new cell divisions in the region of a wound that normal cells are converted into tumor cells of the most rapidly growing type, thus implicating a specific stage (perhaps mitosis) in the normal cell cycle. The initiation of new cell divisions resulting from irritation accompanying a wound has also been found to be essential if tumors are to develop in certain other neoplastic diseases of plants such as Black's wound tumor disease, which is caused by an RNA-containing virus (69), and the Kostoff genetic tumors which arise in certain hybrids within the genus Nicotiana (tobacco) (70).

Similarly, tumor cell transformations resulting from X-irradiation (71), carcinogenic chemicals (72), and viruses

(73) in the animal field have been found to require one or more cell divisions to firmly fix the transformed state in those cell types.

While there doubtless are different specific reasons why cells must proceed through a cell cycle in the different experimental test systems described above if the tumorous state is to be fixed in cells, the important thing that all of these and other systems have in common is that new cell divisions program the genetic information present in a cell for the pattern of metabolism concerned with cell growth and division and, once established, that pattern is firmly and persistently fixed in the cell as a result of the conversion of a normal cell into a tumor cell.

Since the three different plant tumor cell lines, the very slowly growing, the moderately fast growing, and the fast growing, retained indefinitely in culture their characteristic growth patterns, they were admirably suited and were used for a study of the factors required for the rapid autonomous growth of a plant tumor cell (65) (see Fig. 12). In those studies the rapidly growing, fully autonomous tumor cell was used as the standard. That cell type can obviously synthesize all of the essential growth factors and other substances required for its continued rapid growth from the mineral salts, sugar, and three vitamins present in the basic culture medium. The moderately fast growing tumor line required that the basic culture medium be supplemented with the cell enlargement hormone auxin as well as with glutamine and inositol to achieve a growth rate comparable to that of the rapidly growing cell line on the basic culture medium. The very slowly growing tumor line required that the culture medium be supplemented not only with auxin, glutamine, and inositol but with asparagine as well as with a purine and a pyrimidine to achieve a rapid rate of growth. Normal cells do not grow on the basic culture medium. Thus, although the difference between the three types of tumor cells appears to be a quantitative difference since all three types of tumor cells grow indefinitely although at different rates on the basic culture medium, the difference between the three lines of tumor cells and the normal cells is a qualitative difference. A study of the nutritional requirements for the rapid growth of normal cells showed that they were the same as those for the rapid growth of the most slowly growing tumor line with one exception. The normal cells possessed an absolute exogenous requirement for a cell-division-promoting factor. All three tumor cell lines had acquired, as a result of their conversion to tumor cells, an ability to produce that factor. This, then, would appear to represent an essential biochemical difference between the normal cells and the tumor cells since the continued production of that factor by the tumor cells keeps those cells dividing persistently.

The results of this study show us, then, that during the transition from a normal plant cell to a rapidly growing, fully autonomous tumor cell a series of quite distinct but well defined biosynthetic systems, which represent the entire area of metabolism concerned with cell growth and division, become progressively and persistently activated and the degree of activation of those biosynthetic systems within a tumor cell determines the rate of growth of that cell type. The biosynthetic systems that have been shown to be persistently activated in the tumor cells can be divided operationally into two groups. In the first group are the auxin and the cell division factor. These two essential growth-regulating substances establish the pattern of metabolism that is concerned with cell growth and division. Since these two substances are synthesized persistently by the plant tumor cells they maintain that pattern of synthesis in those cells. It is those two essential growth-regulating substances that remove all of the arrest points in the normal cell cycle and, since those two substances are synthesized persistently by the tumor cells, remove the blocks persistently. The other essential substances shown to be produced by the tumor cells are required for the production of essential proteins, nucleic acids and, in the case of inositol, the membrane systems in those cells. Those substances permit the pattern of synthesis established in a cell by the auxin and the cell-division-promoting factor to be expressed.

The development of a capacity by a plant tumor cell for unrestrained or autonomous growth thus finds its explanation in the fact that the tumor cells have acquired a capacity to synthesize persistently all of the essential substances that their normal counterparts require for cell growth and division but cannot themselves make.

Since the plant tumor cells acquire a capacity for autonomous growth as a result of the persistent activation of normally repressed biosynthetic systems, the question that arises is how are these biosynthetic systems persistently activated in the tumor cells. While the entire answer to that question is by no means yet in hand, experimental studies have shown that during the transition from a normal plant cell to a fully autonomous, rapidly growing tumor cell progressive changes occur in the permeability of the membranes that surround the cells (74-76). This increased permeability permits the tumor cells to take up specific inorganic ions and organic solutes very efficiently from the culture medium in which the cells are grown. Specific inorganic ions have been found, moreover, to fully activate most but not quite all of the essential biosynthetic systems found to be functional in the plant tumor cell (see Fig. 14). These differences in the properties of the membrane systems of normal and tumor cells would appear to be of fundamental nature since they permit the activation by inorganic ions of biosynthetic systems that are importantly involved in establishing a capacity for autonomous growth in plant tumor cells. Striking increases in an ability of certain animal tumor cells to take up solutes from the culture medium in which such cells are grown have also been observed (77-80).

The two plant growth-regulating substances are involved not only in removing the arrest points in the normal cell cycle but they also appear to be importantly concerned in determining the rate of growth of plant cells as well as the type of growth that is obtained. Thus, when the concentration of auxin is varied in the presence of a constant amount of cell-division-promoting factor in an otherwise suitable culture medium, the rate of growth of the normal cells is determined by the concentration of auxin in the medium (see Fig. 15). When, on the other hand, the concentration of the cell-division-promoting factor in the medium is high as compared to the concentration of auxin, then the tissue has a tendency to organize shoots and resembles, superficially at least, the complex tumors or teratomas that will be discussed in some

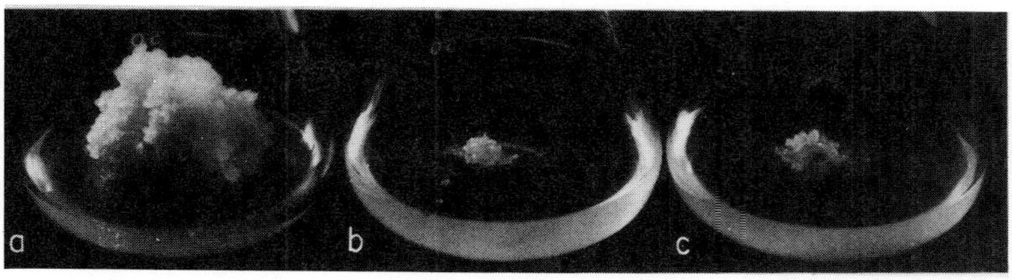


(a) Fast growing tumor line on basic medium

(b) Slow growing tumor line on basic medium

(c) Slow growing tumor line on basic medium + auxin

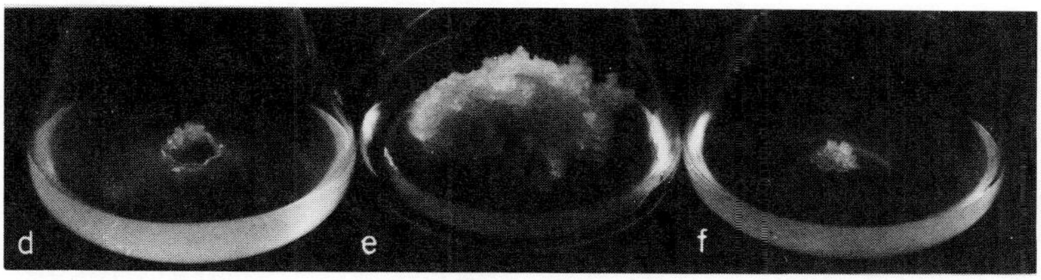


(d) Slow growing tumor line on basic medium in which conc. of four inorganic ions was raised

(e) Slow growing tumor line on basic medium to which auxin has been added and conc. of four inorganic ions raised

(f) Cells stimulated to rapid growth as shown in E transferred to basic medium. Note growth again slows

FIGURE 14. An experiment illustrating the effect of four inorganic ions (K, $NH_3$, $PO_4$, and $NO_3$) on the growth of plant tumor cells. Note a rapidly growing tumor line (a) proliferates actively on a basic culture medium while the very slow growing line (b) grows poorly on that same medium. However, when the concentration of four inorganic ions is raised in the basic culture medium and the medium is supplemented with an auxin, the normally slow growing tumor line grows as rapidly as does the fast growing line on the basic culture medium. Neither auxin alone nor an increased concentration of the four ions in the basic culture medium alone greatly influences the growth rate of the slowly growing tumor line. It is thus possible to replace all of the organic requirements except auxin (see Fig. 12) for rapid growth of the normally slow growing tumor line by raising the concentration of four inorganic ions in the basic culture medium.

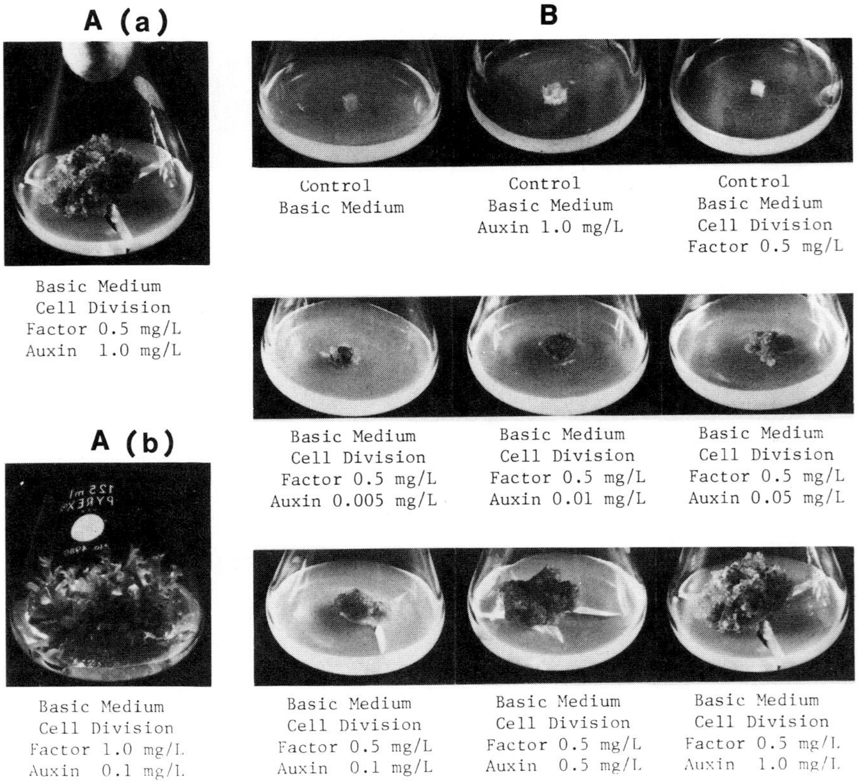


FIGURE 15. The effect of the ratio of an auxin and a cell division factor on growth patterns of normal tobacco pith tissues in culture. A(a), When the ratio of auxin to cell division factor is large, rapidly growing unorganized tissues develop. A(b), When the ratio of cell division factor to auxin is large, tissues that organize shoots develop. (Compare with tumor tissues shown in Fig. 20.) B, The effects on growth rates of normal pith tissues of different concentrations of auxin in the presence of a constant amount of a cell division factor. (Compare with tumor tissues shown in Figs. 11 and 12.) These studies provide a clue to why plant tumor cells grow in an unorganized manner or as teratomatous growths and why such cells grow slowly or proliferate rapidly. In contrast to plant tumor cells, growth of the artificially stimulated normal pith cells does not occur when the two essential growth-regulating substances are absent from the culture medium.

detail later. It is thus possible to reproduce under precisely defined conditions of culture and with the use of normal cells the several types of growth patterns that are found in plant tumor tissues. These studies provide an important clue to why plant tumor cells grow fast or slowly and why they grow in an unorganized or organized manner. The artificially stimulated normal cells are, however, self-limiting and when the externally supplied growth-regulating substances are absent from the medium their growth promptly stops. Plant tumor tissues are, on the other hand, autonomous and are themselves capable of producing all of the growth factors needed for their continued growth both in a host and under completely defined conditions of culture.

## DEVELOPMENT OF AUTONOMY IN ANIMAL CELLS

Can the concept of autonomy that has been developed for plant tumor systems be made to serve as models for animal tumor systems as well? It is clear that success in characterizing the nature of autonomy in plant tumor systems depended largely on the development and use of a selective culture medium that permitted the active proliferation of tumor cells but not of comparable normal cell types and thus to reproduce in cell culture the situation that occurs in a host. This same strategy has recently been applied to an animal tumor system in an attempt to gain insight into the basic cellular mechanisms that underlie autonomy in that system (81) (see Fig. 16). An attempt was made in that study to reproduce as closely as possible in cell culture the conditions that are known to exist in an animal host. In that study blood plasma was used in place of blood serum. Although serum is almost universally used in animal cell and tissue culture studies and is known to contain substances that stimulate cell divisions, it is not serum but blood plasma that normally nourishes cells in animals. Freshly isolated cells rather than established cell lines were used in that study because many significant changes in the properties of cells may occur as a consequence of their prolonged growth in culture. An experimental system was also used in these studies in which virtually all of the normal cells in the culture medium could be transformed into tumor cells in short periods of time. These criteria were largely satisfied by using fibroblasts obtained from pectoral muscles of young adult chickens. The fibroblasts were isolated and passaged twice in culture and then divided into two groups. One of these groups of cells was transformed into tumor cells with the Schmidt-Ruppin strain of the Rous sarcoma virus while the other group was used as the normal control cells. When these two groups of cells were grown

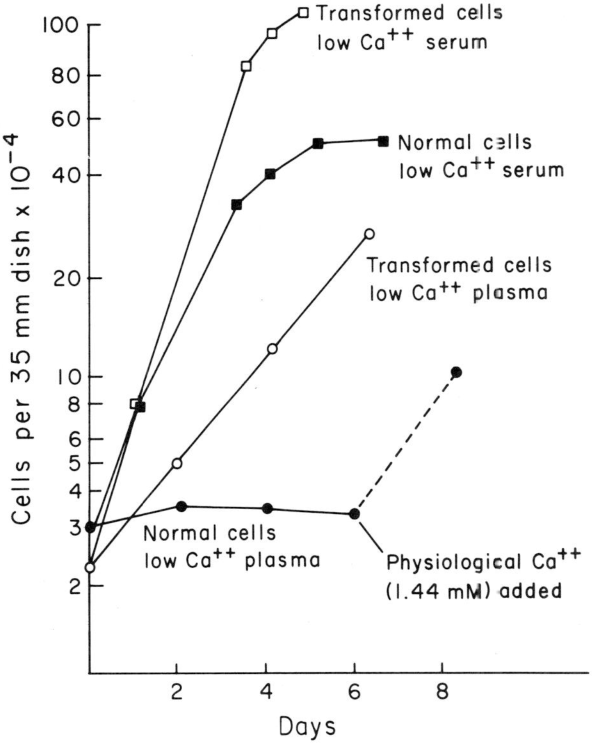


FIGURE 16. Growth of normal chicken fibroblasts and Rous sarcoma virus-transformed fibroblasts plated in culture media supplemented with either serum or plasma obtained from the same lot of blood and containing either physiological concentrations of the $Ca^{++}$ ion or very low concentrations of that ion. Note that the transformed cells proliferate actively in a low $Ca^{++}$ plasma-containing medium while the normal cells remain essentially quiescent under those conditions of culture. The resting normal cells can be made to proliferate actively either by adding physiological concentrations of $Ca^{++}$ to the low $Ca^{++}$ plasma-containing medium or by substituting serum for plasma in the low $Ca^{++}$ medium. Growth of the normal fibroblasts appears therefore to be regulated by some $Ca^{++}$-mediated function and this essential function can be replaced by one or more factors present in serum.

separately in a conventional serum-containing medium containing either normal concentrations of the $Ca^{++}$ ions or low concentrations of that ion, both normal cells and tumor cells proliferated actively. When, however, blood plasma was substituted for serum in a low $Ca^{++}$-containing culture medium the tumor cells proliferated actively while the normal cells, although maintained, remained essentially quiescent. It was thus possible to reproduce in cell culture the situation as it is found to occur in a host in which the tumor cells proliferate actively while the growth of the normal cells is precisely regulated. It was found, further, that when the normal fibroblasts were maintained in an essentially resting state for three or more days in the low $Ca^{++}$ plasma medium and then either serum was substituted for plasma in the low $Ca^{++}$ medium or the concentration of the $Ca^{++}$ ion was raised to physiological levels in the plasma-containing medium, the normal cells proliferated actively. The amount of growth obtained with the normal cells reflected, moreover, the concentration of the $Ca^{++}$ ion in the plasma-containing culture medium. The results of this study indicate, then, that growth of the normal fibroblasts is regulated by some as yet uncharacterized $Ca^{++}$ ion-mediated function and that growth of the cancerous fibroblasts results either from an increased ability of the tumor cells to take up the $Ca^{++}$ ion from very dilute solution or from an alteration or bypass of that $Ca^{++}$-mediated function in the tumor cells. It was found, further, that the $Ca^{++}$ ion functioned by initiating some critical reaction in the G1 phase of the cell cycle and that once this function had been activated it set into operation the necessarily complex series of reactions that led to the duplication of the chromosomal DNA, mitosis, and, finally, to cell divisions.

That the $Ca^{++}$ ion plays a most important role in regulating the normal cell division cycle is evidenced by the fact that a wide variety of cell types which include, in addition to chicken fibroblasts (81, 82), human peripheral lymphocytes, rat bone marrow cells, heart cells, liver cells, thymic lymphoblasts, among others, are controlled by that ion (83). In all of these instances, as in the case of the chicken fibroblasts, the $Ca^{++}$ ion functions by removing the block for cell division that exists in the G1 phase of the cell cycle. It has now been reported, moreover, that a number of different malignant tumors which are caused by diverse chemical and biological agents proliferate actively in a low $Ca^{++}$ ion medium as do the tumorous chicken fibroblasts. These include a rhabdomyosarcoma that was induced in rat thigh muscle with nickel sulfide (84), as well as three different mouse tumors one of which was initiated by the cancer-producing chemical methylcholanthrene, the second by the RNA-containing murine sarcoma virus, while the third was induced by the DNA-containing simian vacuolating virus (SV40) (85).

Since all of the diverse tumor cell types thus far tested have been found to proliferate actively in a $Ca^{++}$-deficient medium that does not support the growth of comparable normal cells, it has been suggested that this property may ultimately prove to be a reliable indicator for the neoplastic transformation (85).

Although the precise role that the $Ca^{++}$ ion plays in removing the G1 phase block in the normal cell cycle is not yet known with certainty, several possible ways in which that ion may be implicated have been suggested (85, 86). A calcium-dependent regulatory protein has, moreover, now been identified in normal and virally transformed chicken fibroblasts (87). Although significantly greater levels of this protein were found in virally transformed cells than in normal resting cells, intermediate levels of the modulator protein were found in dividing normal cells. The results of this study would suggest, then, that elevated levels of the $Ca^{++}$-dependent protein are associated with the growth process rather than with transformation *per se*.

It has recently been suggested, without support of experimental evidence, that the $Ca^{++}$ ion may be acting indirectly to promote cell growth and division through competition with the $Mg^{++}$ ion for membrane sites, thereby making the released $Mg^{++}$ ion available for otherwise rate-limiting chemical (transphorylation) reactions (88). While this may possibly be found to be one function of the $Ca^{++}$ ion it is clearly not the only one or even the main one and other of its more specific roles in regulating the cell cycle have been discussed in detail elsewhere (83). This does not, of course, mean that the $Mg^{++}$ ion may not also play an important regulatory role. It has, in fact, now been found that the $Mg^{++}$ ion is an essential cofactor which is required for the activity of the cytoplasmic initiator of chromosomal DNA synthesis and thus clearly plays a role in the removal of the G1 phase block in the normal cell cycle (62).

Since specific inorganic ions play a most important role in the regulation of cell growth and division in both the animal and plant fields, the results reported above appear to represent a start in the right direction. If these findings are now explored further they could well provide meaningful insight into those changes in proliferative behavior that constitute the ultimate basis of the tumor problem generally.

An interesting observation that has been studied only in a very limited way suggests that differences in sensitivity of certain normal cells and comparable tumor cells to starvation may exist. If certain normal cells (baby hamster kidney cells) are placed in a culture medium from which an essential nutrient (e.g., glutamine or isoleucine) is absent, growth of the cells stops and they are all arrested in the same stage of the cell cycle. If virally transformed hamster cells are similarly starved, growth of those cells will also eventually stop but, unlike the normal cells, growth of the tumor cells is not arrested at a specific stage in the cell cycle but those cells are blocked at different stages as though they had randomly run out of an essential nutrient. If, now, after a starvation period of 63 hours, the essential nutrient is restored to the culture medium, growth of the normal cells begins almost immediately while growth of the transformed cells does not. It was found that the virally transformed cells had been killed when incubated for 63 hours in the starvation medium while the normal cells had not. The results of those studies suggest, then, that striking differences in sensitivity to starvation exist between normal cells and tumor cells in the hamster system at least. If further studies show that this observation has broader application it may prove useful for the selective killing of tumor cells (89, 90).

## CAPACITY OF CANCER CELLS TO INVADE AND METASTASIZE

In addition to the development of a capacity of all true tumor cells to proliferate in an essentially unrestrained or autonomous manner in their hosts, malignant cells are characterized by an ability to invade underlying normal tissues and to detach small groups of cells from the tumor which then move or metastasize through the blood vessels and lymph channels where new tumors may arise. It was pointed out earlier that the development of a capacity to grow autonomously, to invade and metastasize are dissociable characters which may be inherited independently of one another. The ability of cells to invade and move freely through an organism is not, moreover, limited to malignant cells since these properties may be expressed by certain normal cell types as well. For example, the active migration of certain normal cells plays an important role in the structural molding of a developing embryo. Cells known as melanoblasts migrate actively through many tissues of an embryo before finally becoming localized at specific sites, after which they differentiate into non-migrating melanocytes. Similarly, certain normal white blood cells such as the macrophages, leukocytes, and lymphocytes invade normal tissues extensively and move freely through an organism. These migrating cells thus show certain fundamental attributes of malignant cells but, in their normal state, lack a capacity for autonomous growth. Since all normal cells, with very few exceptions, contain a complete complement of genes and since certain genes code for the cellular properties that lead to a capacity of cells to invade and metastasize, it would appear reasonable to assume that the abilities to invade and metastasize are inherently present but not expressed, at least not to the same degree, in most if not all normal cells. If that is true then it should be possible to cause normal cells to develop for the time being as do malignant cells by treating them with appropriate substances that do not in themselves transform normal cells into tumor cells. That this can, in fact, be done was demonstrated shortly after the turn of the prssent century (91). It was found in that study that when the red dye Scharlach R was injected under the skin of rabbits' ears the epithelial cells that were in intimate contact with the dye multiplied actively, invaded underlying normal tissues deeply and even entered the blood vessels and lymph channels. Although these stimulated normal cells mimic perfectly the malignant state, they revert to normal when the dye disappears from the site of injection. The results of studies such as those described above suggest, then, that all of the genetic information necessary to establish the malignant state is present in normal epithelial cells and the problem appears to resolve itself into learning how that information is persistently activated, a matter that was considered earlier.

More recent studies have shown that a factor, known as the "overgrowth stimulating factor," is produced by virally transformed chicken fibroblasts which when isolated and applied to normal fibroblasts in culture causes those cells to behave for the time being as though they were tumorous (92). Since trypsin and pronase, when applied to normal fibroblasts in culture, could reproduce perfectly the effects of the "overgrowth stimulating factor" it seems likely that that factor is a proteolytic enzyme.

Proteolytic enzymes probably influence the growth of cells by altering the surface properties of cells and, more particularly, the properties of the surface membranes. We now have clues to how those enzymes may act to affect changes in the cellular membranes. Before considering this matter further we should perhaps digress briefly and attempt to identify the evidence upon which is based the belief that differences exist in the surface properties of normal cells and malignant cells. That such differences exist is evidenced by the fact that many animal cancer cells and particularly the more malignant cells are held loosely together and are much more easily separated from one another by mechanical means than are comparable normal cells or cells present in benign tumors. It has been suggested that reduced adhesiveness shown by malignant cells may constitute the physical basis of malignancy (93). Reduced "stickiness" shown by malignant cells is evidenced further by the observation that when normal cells and tumor cells are grown in culture they may show striking differences in their movements and behavior. When, for example, normal fibroblasts are plated in a conventional culture medium containing 10 percent serum the cells move actively, and when two or more cells come in contact they tend to adhere to one another and line up in parallel fashion. Such cells commonly grow until they reach a confluent monolayer after which time growth stops (see Fig. 17). The normal cells must, moreover, be plated on a surface to which they can attach and spread out if they are to multiply actively. Malignant cells often behave quite differently under similar conditions of culture. The growth of those cells is less coordinated, is not contact inhibited, and the cells move freely over one another in random fashion (see Fig. 17). Unlike normal cells, the malignant cells are not anchorage-dependent for growth and they may even proliferate actively when suspended in a liquid or semisolid culture medium. The saturation density reached by malignant cells in culture is commonly greater than that of normal cells grown under similar conditions (see Fig. 16).

If the observed differences in the behavior of normal cells and malignant cells are, in fact, due to differences in the surface properties of those cells, then it should be possible to characterize more specifically differences that exist in the two cell types.

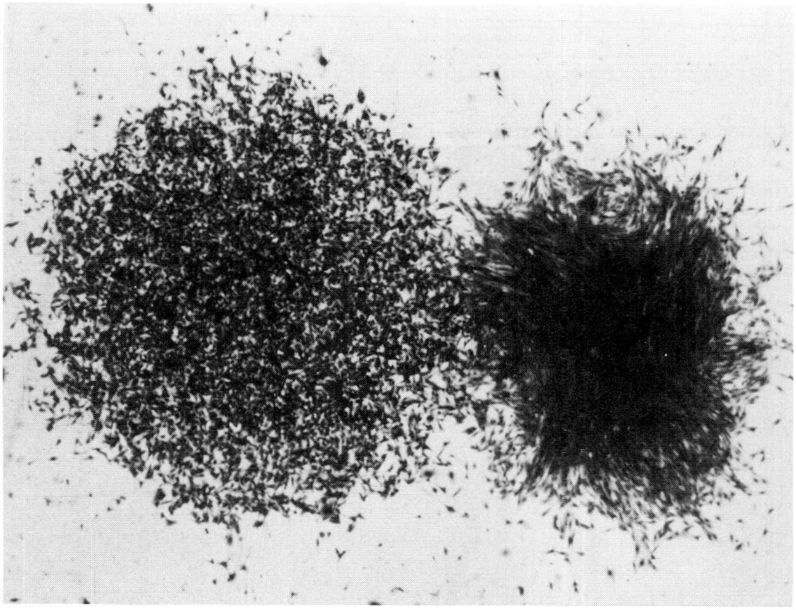

FIGURE 17. Picture of colonies of hamster cells showing (left) the tumor phenotype and (right) the normal phenotype. Note that cells showing the normal phenotype are lined up in parallel array while those showing the tumor phenotype grow randomly. The colony at the right was derived from cells transformed by the Rous sarcoma virus and that had reverted spontaneously from the tumor to the normal phenotype. (Courtesy of Dr. Ian Macpherson)

Membranes that line the surface of cells are not mere passive barriers but are complex, highly ordered, and dynamic structures. They have sometimes been described as being "islands of proteins floating in a sea of lipids." Among the substances present in membranes are enzymes and other proteins, glycoproteins (proteins that contain sugars), glycolipids, phospholipids, etc. Of these the glycoproteins appear particularly interesting as far as the present discussion is concerned. It has been found that membranes of normal resting cells contain a glycoprotein known as the large external transformation-sensitive protein, LETS for short. This protein is found to be present in far smaller amounts in membranes of actively dividing normal cells and to be essentially absent in membranes of tumor cells. Normal cells growing in culture deposit a residue which is known as the substrate attached material, or SAM, and which is composed partly of LETS protein. Malignant cells do not produce this protein. Of interest is the finding that when the SAM protein is added to a culture of tumor cells those cells grow for the time being in an essentially normal manner. The membranes of the transformed cells thus seem to lack adequate amounts of the LETS glycoprotein and this, in turn, appears somehow to influence their growth.

Differences in the surface properties of normal and

malignant cells may be manifested in other ways. Many cancer cells clump or agglutinate when treated with specially prepared plant proteins that are known as lectins (see Fig. 18). Although there are many different kinds of lectins, the two most commonly used for experimental work are known as concanavalin A (obtained from jack beans) and wheat germ agglutinin. Some of the earlier studies showed that cancer cells agglutinate readily in the presence of smaller amounts of lectin than do normal cells. However, when normal cells are

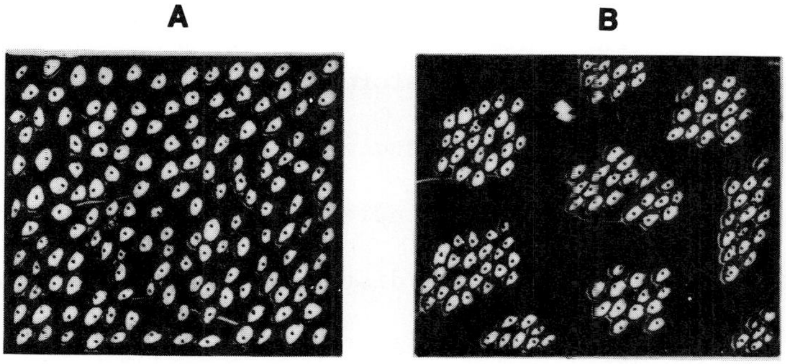


FIGURE 18. Drawings illustrate differences in the response of (A) normal (hamster) cells and (B) virally transformed hamster cells to the lectin concanavalin A. Normal cells in suspension do not commonly clump or agglutinate when treated with lectins such as concanavalin A. However, shortly after they become transformed to tumor cells they clump when treated with the same concentration of lectin that does not affect normal cells. These findings indicate that changes occur at the surface of the cells following transformation.

treated with a proteolytic enzyme such as trypsin they may agglutinate as readily as do cancer cells when both are treated with concanavalin A (94-96). Consistent differences were found to exist, moreover, between the binding of lectin and the normal and tumor phenotype in temperature-sensitive SV40-transformed 3T3 cells. Thus, when transformed cells were grown at 32°C and showed the tumor phenotype they bound significantly more of the lectin than when incubated at 39°C and showed the normal phenotype (97). The binding sites on normal and tumor cells appear, therefore, to be similar and it has been suggested that the difference in agglutinability of the two cell types reflects a redistribution of those sites in the membranes during transformation (98).

The results of recent studies using another temperature-sensitive viral system have indicated that concanavalin A receptor sites are uniformly distributed in the membranes of cells that show the normal phenotype and they do not become clustered upon addition of a lectin. In contrast, the receptor sites for concanavalin A in cells that show the tumor phenotype are mobile and become clustered in the membrane when treated with the lectin and the cells then agglutinate. Whether the receptor sites for concanavalin A remain uniformly distributed in the membranes or become clustered has been correlated with the ordered or disordered state of a specific protein which is similar to a protein responsible for muscle contraction. This protein is present in the form of sheaths and forms part of the skeleton of a cell. Thus, when cells show the normal phenotype this contractile protein is in an ordered state and the receptor sites for the lectin are uniformly distributed in the membranes, while an increase in mobility of the receptor sites occurs when the transformed state is expressed and this is correlated with a disordering of the protein sheaths (99). It has been found, moreover, that when normal cells are treated with certain proteolytic enzymes the protein sheaths disappear while when transformed cells are treated with specific inhibitors of those enzymes the sheaths reform. Thus, proteolytic enzymes not only influence the membranes directly but also affect the cell skeleton which, in turn, must also influence the properties of the membranes.

It has long been known that lectins can initiate cell division in certain normally resting cell types such as, for example, the lymphocytes. Lectins have therefore been used to study cell growth and division. Concanavalin A has been found to possess four binding sites. By modifying the molecule chemically with succinic acid, two components, each possessing two binding sites, were obtained. This modified molecule was found to bind to receptor sites in the cell membranes but they no longer caused the treated cells to agglutinate. When transformed cells were treated with the modified lectin they again acquired a need to attach to a substrate if they were to grow and divide. They thus behaved in this respect as do normal cells. The plant lectins have been found to be as effective as insulin, through direct interaction with insulin receptors, in enhancing the rate of glucose uptake as well as in other insulin-mediated responses (100). Striking increases in the uptake of certain essential substances from a culture medium by cancer cells have been observed by a number of investigators (77-79). It has been suggested that the growth of cells is controlled by modification of membrane transport sites that regulate the availability of essential nutrients (101).

Differences in surface properties of normal cells and tumor cells may be manifested in other ways. In cancer cells characteristic antigens may be found in the cells or on the surface of the cells. Those found on the surface, like the receptor sites for the lectins, reflect changes in the surface properties of the cell membranes. These new surface antigens, known as transplantation antigens, are particularly interesting because, as we shall see later, they may render tumor cells vulnerable to immunological attack by their hosts.

In addition to such membrane-associated changes in tumor

cells that lead to increased agglutinability with lectins, presence of new surface antigens, alterations in permeability and transport mechanisms there are changes in membrane-associated enzymatic activities. One of these is a membrane-associated proteolytic enzyme known as the plasminogen activator. This enzyme has been found to act on plasminogen, which is a component of the serum in which the cells are grown, to give rise to another proteolytic enzyme, fibrinolysin, which, as the name implies, digests fibrin and certain other proteins (102, 103). It has been reported, moreover, that many tumors show increased concentrations of proteolytic enzymes at or near their most actively growing cells. The growth of cancer cells of several different kinds can be inhibited by a variety of inhibitors of proteolytic enzymes (104). The production of fibrinolysin from plasminogen by the plasminogen activator appears to be more concerned with an ability of malignant cells to invade and metastasize than with an ability of those cells to grow autonomously (105). This suggestion is supported by the observation that while the expression of several phenotypic properties of transformed cells (ability to grow as colonies in soft agar, tumor cell morphology, etc.) requires the presence of serum plasminogen, virally transformed hamster cells grow to high cell densities in a plasminogen-depleted medium (106).

Differences in the ability of normal cells and cancer cells to migrate may be demonstrated directly by a very simple type of experiment which is illustrated in Figure 19. A so-called "migration factor" which could contribute importantly to the malignant state has now been isolated but not yet characterized chemically (107). It was found in that study that when a confluent monolayer of normal cells is wounded by scraping away part of the cell sheet, the normal cells do not migrate into the cleared area unless serum is present in the culture medium. In contrast, malignant cells do migrate into the cleared area in a serum-free medium. A specific "migration factor" was found to be released into a serum-free medium by the malignant cells but not by the normal cell line. Should such a "migration factor" be found to be associated with the malignant state in other cancers but not with the normal or benign states it would, needless to say, have profound implications as far as our understanding of the ability of cancer cells to invade and metastasize is concerned.

It has recently been reported, further, that a contact-inhibited normal cell line produces a specific protein-containing substance which is capable of restoring contact inhibition of growth in a highly malignant cell line (108). Thus, both the capacities for cell migration as well as contact inhibition of growth appear in these instances to

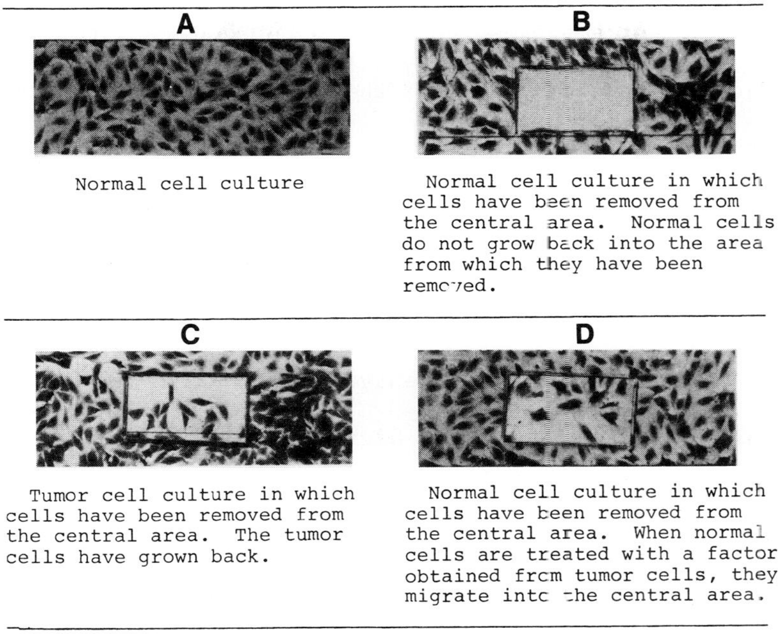


FIGURE 19. Experiment of the type that provides evidence that a migration factor is produced by malignant cells. (A) Confluent monolayer culture of normal hamster cells. When such a culture is wounded by removing part of the cell sheet the normal cells (B) do not migrate into the cleared area unless serum is present in the culture medium, while malignant cells (C) do migrate into the cleared area in a serum-free medium. It has been found (D) that the malignant cells produce a specific protein which when added to normal cells in culture encourages those cells to migrate into the cleared area in a serum-free medium.

be controlled by specific substances.

Although many of the changes that occur at the cell surface during the transition from a normal cell to a malignant cell are poorly understood, the results obtained thus far are sufficiently suggestive to indicate that many cellular properties, including some of the most important ones that distinguish normal cells from cancer cells, may be expressed as surface properties. An understanding of the nature of the changes that occur in the cellular membranes are, nevertheless, important not only because of the insight that they may provide into why cells behave as they do but because certain of those changes are highly specific and thus open possible new avenues of approach for very selectively attacking and destroying cancer cells.

# CHAPTER IV

## NATURE OF THE HERITABLE CELLULAR CHANGE, I.

## EPIGENETIC MECHANISMS

One of the most puzzling aspects of the tumor problem is concerned with the multiplicity of diverse physical, chemical, and biological agents that are capable of converting normal cells into tumor cells. These agencies with the exception of the oncogenic viruses are concerned only with the inception of tumors and play no role in the continued abnormal growth of the tumor cells once the cellular change has been accomplished. As was noted earlier in this discussion, the tumorous state often expresses itself in ways which are independent of causative agents. From a clinical point of view nothing distinguishes tumors produced in experimental animals with radiation, cancer-producing chemicals, or by the oncogenic viruses. There is, moreover, reason to believe that the disease in these instances is the same with the same underlying cause. The implication of this would appear to be that all of the diverse cancer-producing agents ultimately affect a common cellular mechanism which, once deranged, urges the tumor cells to continued abnormal and unrestrained growth in their hosts. If that is true it would suggest that the underlying heritable cellular change found in the diversely initiated tumors ultimately converges at the same point in a cell. Our problem now will be to attempt to identify that hypothetical point.

The fact that the characteristic properties of tumor cells, like genetic traits generally, are faithfully transmitted to their descendants over long periods of time suggests that we must turn our attention first to the genetic material present in a cell because, as we have seen, most if not all traits, whether normal or abnormal, are ultimately determined by that information.

Since the development of the tumorous state represents an abnormal condition, it would appear that either something drastic has happened to the integrity of some of the genetic information and/or that all of the essential genetic information is present in a tumor cell but that something has gone wrong with the regulation of that information. A distinction between changes in the integrity of the genetic information present in a tumor cell and persistent changes in the expression of that information would appear to be of more than just academic interest. If changes of a mutational type involving the loss, replacement, or permanent rearrangement of the genetic information are involved in establishing the tumorous state, then it implies that the heritable cellular change is of a permanent and irreversible type. The concept of irreversibility of the tumorous state had, in fact, dominated the thinking of cancer biologists for many years. If, on the other hand, persistent changes in the expression of the genetic information underlie the tumorous state, then the process is potentially reversible and offers, in principle at least, entirely new avenues of approach to the tumor problem.

Possible cellular mechanisms that involve a change in the integrity of the genetic information present in a cell and that could, in principle at least, account for the continued abnormal and autonomous proliferation of a tumor cell may be listed as follows: (*A*) loss of some of the genetic information; (*B*) mutations resulting from base-pair substitutions in the chromosomal DNA; (*C*) mutations of a frameshift type; (*D*) the translocation of some of the genetic information present in a cell leading to a permanent rearrangement of some of that information; (*E*) qualitative or quantitative changes in the balance of chromosomes or chromosome parts due to nondisjunction, aneuploidy, or polyploidy; and (F) addition and integration of new genetic information into the genome of a cell resulting from infection by the cancer-producing viruses.

The question that we must now consider is whether a profound and heritable change in the phenotype of a cell can occur without a corresponding change in the integrity of the genetic information that is present in a cell. If the answer to that question is in the negative, then tumorigenesis must clearly involve one or more of the mechanisms described above. If, on the other hand, an affirmative answer can be provided experimentally, then quite different mechanisms can be envisioned for the origin of a tumor cell.

Persistent but potentially reversible changes in the phenotype of a cell without corresponding changes in the integrity of the genetic information present in the cell have been described for many different organisms (109, 110). The diversity of cellular mechanisms that may underlie such heritable cellular changes is well illustrated in the case of the protozoon *Paramecium*. Here we find (A) the so-called "killer phenomenon" which is dependent on the presence in the cells of kappa particles which, in turn, represent DNA-containing parasites (111); (B) the Dauermodifications of Jollos which are concerned with the inheritance of acquired tolerance to certain toxic substances (112); (C) the alternative serotypes (113) and mating types (114) found in that protozoon; and (D) cytotaxis or cortical inheritance which is largely determined by pre-existing structure (115). One of the most commonly found types of persistent but potentially reversible heritable cellular changes in the phenotype of a cell without a corresponding change in the integrity of the genome is that which accompanies cellular differentiation that occurs during the normal course of development in all higher organisms.

Our problem now will be to attempt to determine which one or more, if any, of the different types of genetic or epigenetic mechanisms listed above is most likely to underlie the tumorous state generally. In attempting to resolve the questions raised above we might begin by asking whether there is any experimental evidence to show that the tumorous state may, in fact, be initiated and maintained in the presence of a complete and unaltered complement of host cell genes. The fact that a significant number of tumors have now been found to have an essentially normal complement of chromosomes suggests that all of the genetic information may be retained in cells of those tumors. The fact, as was discussed earlier, that certain normal cell types may temporarily show one or more or all of the essential properties that characterize the malignant state (e.g., unrestrained growth, ability to invade and metastasize) in the presence of appropriate stimuli (Scharlach R) suggests, moreover, that all of the genetic information necessary to establish the cancer phenotype is present in normal epithelial cells and that the maintenance of the cancerous state is merely a question of determining how that information is regulated so that it is persistently expressed in those cell types. The ultimate proof that normal cells contain all of the genetic information required for the establishment and maintenance of the tumorous state would be provided by a demonstration that that state can be achieved in the absence of the addition, deletion, or permanent rearrangement of genetic information normally present in a cell and that once that state is firmly fixed as a heritable cellular trait it is completely reversible, leading again to normal cells of the type from which the tumor was derived. Examples of this are now available in both the plant and the animal literature and select tumor systems will be described to illustrate the reversibility of the tumorous state.

## REVERSAL OF THE TUMOROUS STATE IN PLANTS

### Habituation

When normal cells are isolated from a plant and grown for prolonged periods in culture they may acquire, as do animal cells, tumorous properties. In plants this phenomenon is known as habituation and results, as we have seen, from a persistent activation of specific biosynthetic systems the products of which are concerned with cell growth and division. These essential biosynthetic systems may be activated individually or more than one may become persistently activated more or less simultaneously. When, for example, the biosynthetic system that produces the cell-division-promoting factor is persistently activated without a corresponding activation of the auxin system, then the resulting cells behave as conditional or hormone-dependent tumor cells in that such cells must be continually provided with an exogenous source of the plant hormone auxin but not with a cell division factor if growth accompanied by cell division is to occur (116). When, on the other hand, all of the essential biosynthetic systems are persistently activated in habituated cells they behave as do true plant tumor cells. These newly acquired properties may be retained indefinitely. This, then, represents a heritable cellular change that is highly stable and occurs spontaneously in the absence of any recognizable tumor-producing agent. That habituation is completely reversible under special conditions has now been demonstrated experimentally (116, 117). A demonstration of the reversibility of the tumorous state was possible in this instance only because of certain unique properties possessed by higher plant species. The first of these is that cells of higher plants may be totipotential, that is, an entirely normal, fully fertile plant may be obtained from a single somatic cell which may be of a specialized type. The second property possessed by higher plant species is the unique way in which they grow. Primary growth results from the very rapid division, subsequent elongation and, finally, the differentiation of cells at the extreme apex of a shoot or a root. By making use of these two properties it was possible to achieve not only a recovery from the tumorous state in the case of habituated tissues but of certain other plant tumor systems as well. In the case of habituation, single habituated cells were isolated and grown separately in culture. These grew as typical tumor cells on a basic culture medium and they retained their tumorous properties. When, however, the progeny of those single cells were planted on a special inductive medium they organized tumor shoots, and when such shoots were isolated and grown further they ultimately recovered from the tumorous state and gave rise to plants that flowered and set viable seed. When such seed was sown it gave rise to plants that had recovered from the tumorous state. Since the phenomenon of habituation is completely reversible under special experimental conditions, the results obtained in these studies provide the ultimate proof that the tumorous state in plants may arise and be perpetuated indefinitely in the absence of the addition, deletion, or permanent rearrangement of essential genetic material present in a normal cell. All of the genetic material required to establish and maintain the tumorous state is present in the genome of the normal cell and whether the tumor phenotype or the normal phenotype is expressed is determined by which of the genes are functional and which are repressed.

## The Crown Gall Disease

A second tumorous disease that has been shown to be reversible is the crown gall disease of plants. This disease, as was indicated earlier, is initiated by a tumor-inducing principle (TIP) that is transmitted to plant cells by a specific bacterium. The TIP, which appears to be a plasmid carried by the bacteria, is capable of regularly converting normal plant cells into tumor cells in short periods of time.

Once the cellular change has occurred the continued abnormal and autonomous proliferation of the tumor cells becomes an automatic process that is entirely independent of the bacteria. It was found that when totipotential cells present in a plant such as, for example, tobacco are transformed into tumor cells there results, in place of a characteristic tumor, a complex overgrowth or teratoma. Such teratomas are composed of a chaotic assembly of tissues and organs that may be very abnormal in appearance. When tumor cells were isolated from the abnormal but organized structures that developed from the teratomas and planted on a basic culture medium, those cells proliferated actively on that medium as did typical crown gall tumor cells. The basic medium did not support the growth of normal cells of the type from which the tumor cells were derived. The teratoma-derived tumor cells differ from typical crown gall tumor cells in that they may retain indefinitely in culture a capacity to organize tumor shoots (see Fig. 20). That these teratoma tissues were composed entirely of tumor cells and not a mixture of normal cells and tumor cells was demonstrated by isolating single cells and showing that the progeny of these single tumor cells retained a capacity to organize tumor shoots. When such tumor shoots that were derived from and were the progeny of a single teratoma cell were isolated from the tissues and grafted to

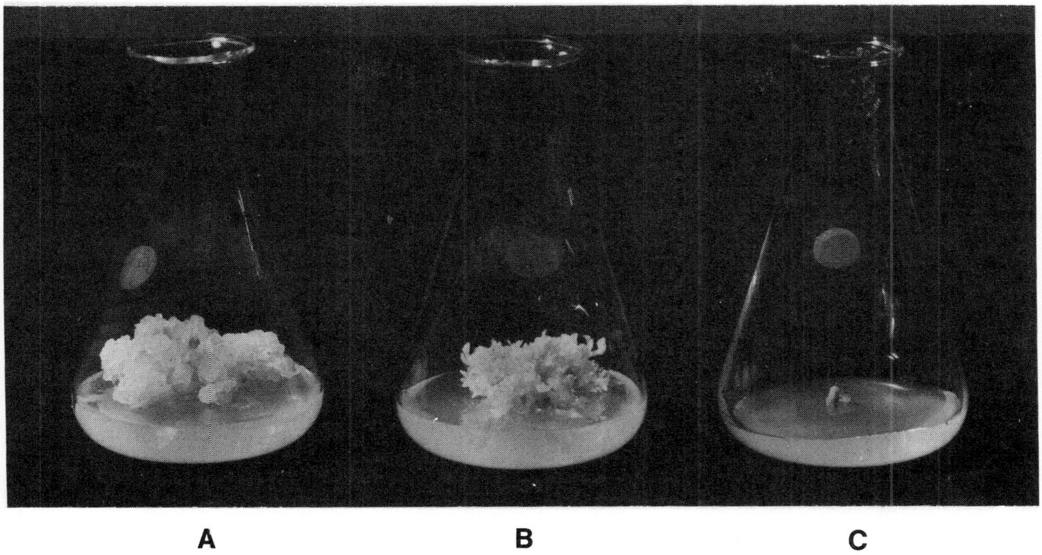


FIGURE 20. Growth patterns of (A) typical unorganized crown gall tumor tissue grown on a basic culture medium, (B) crown gall teratoma tissue, and (C) normal tissue. Note that teratoma tissue retains a capacity to organize tumor buds and shoots.

the cut stem tip of an appropriate plant a wide spectrum of responses was observed. Under the best conditions the teratoma-derived shoots developed quite normally and some of these ultimately flowered and set viable seed. When those seeds were sown they gave rise to typical tobacco plants the cells of which were no longer tumorous (118-120). Thus a complete recovery from the tumorous state had been achieved. These studies demonstrate then that all of the genetic information necessary to reconstitute an entirely normal plant may be retained by the plant tumor cells over long periods of time in culture.

A second phenomenon, one concerned with the suppression of the tumorous state rather than a recovery from that state, is also illustrated with the use of this experimental test system (119). As was indicated when the teratoma shoots are grafted to appropriate host plants, some of these develop quite normally and the leaves that develop on such shoots appear normal. Those teratoma-derived leaves contain all of the specialized cell types found in normal leaves and those cells have been found to be fully functional. The cells of such teratoma-derived leaves are clearly not showing tumorous properties and appear by all generally accepted criteria to be normal. Yet it was found that when the specialized cell types that were present in the teratoma-derived leaves were isolated and grown in culture they again assumed their tumorous properties. The results of that study demonstrated, then, that the substances and mechanisms that govern so precisely the growth, cellular differentiation, and organ formation during the normal course of development of a higher organism are also operative in directing the development of the teratoma shoots. The specialized cell types present in the teratoma leaves need only to be released from the restraining mechanisms present in an intact organism to again assume their tumorous properties. Thus we see that while a persistent but potentially reversible suppression of the tumorous state is a characteristic feature of the vegetative phase of teratoma shoot growth, a recovery from that state occurs during the reproductive phase. An analysis of the reproductive process has now shown that a recovery from the tumorous state occurs at meiosis rather than during later stages of sexual reproduction (120). A composite picture illustrating the suppression of and a recovery from the tumorous state in the crown gall disease is shown in Figure 21. See also reference 120a.

## REVERSAL OF THE TUMOROUS STATE IN ANIMALS

### Teratocarcinoma of the Mouse

The question that arises next is whether this sort of thing is unique to plant tumor systems or whether it occurs in animal tumors as well. Is, in other words, all of the essential genetic information present in a normal animal cell conserved when that cell is transformed into a cancer cell or is it necessary to postulate drastic changes of a mutational type in the genetic information to account for the development of the cancerous state? This question can perhaps best be answered with the use of a number of specific examples which have been selected for discussion because they illustrate the

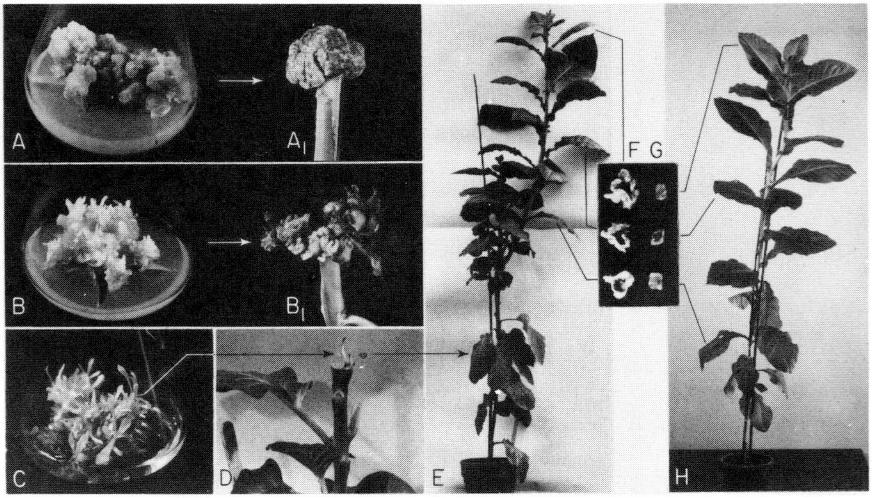


FIGURE 21. A composite picture illustrating the suppression of and a recovery from the tumorous state in the crown gall disease of plants. (A) Typical unorganized crown gall tumor tissue. (A1) Growth pattern obtained when a fragment of tissue shown in (A) is grafted to the cut stem tip of a normal plant. (B) Crown gall teratoma tissue. Note this tissue organizes tumor buds and shoots. (B1) Growth pattern obtained when a fragment of tissue shown in (B) is grafted to the cut stem tip of a normal plant. (C) Teratoma tissue shown in (B) grown in a culture medium that encouraged the development of tumor shoots. Tumor shoots such as are shown in (C) were grafted individually to the cut stem tip of a normal tobacco plant (D). Under the best conditions a tumor shoot developed quite normally and ultimately flowered and set viable seed (E). When such seed was sown it gave rise to plants that had recovered from the tumorous state (H). An analysis of leaves and stems of the teratoma-derived shoots pictured in (E) showed that they were composed of all of the specialized cell types found in normal leaves and those cells were fully functional. When those specialized, fully functional leaf cells were isolated and planted on a basic culture medium they again assumed their tumorous properties (F). Similar leaf tissue fragments isolated from a recovered plant (H) did not grow on a basic culture medium. These plants had recovered from the tumorous state. Thus, although a persistent but potentially reversible suppression of the tumorous state is a characteristic feature of the vegetative phase of teratoma shoot growth, a recovery from the tumorous state occurs during the sexual reproductive process and, more particularly, during meiosis.

point that we are attempting to establish.

The first system that we will consider is a malignant teratocarcinoma of the mouse. This cancer, like the plant teratomas described above, is a complex tumor and commonly contains eight to fourteen well-differentiated cell types such as epithelial cells, nerve cells, muscle cells, bone, cartilage, tooth buds, hair follicles, etc., which are scattered in completely disorganized array in the tumor. Interspersed among these well-differentiated cell types are essentially undifferentiated cells which are known as embryonal carcinoma cells. When such tumors are transplanted serially in mice this broad spectrum of cell types is reproduced indefinitely. The question that initially arose in studying this tumor was whether the differentiated cells present in the cancer developed independently or whether they all arose from a common stem cell type. To test the latter hypothesis, single embryonal carcinoma cells were injected into mice. The results of this study showed that in those instances in which the single cancer cells established themselves and grew, malignant tumors developed that killed the mice in a few weeks' time (121). Microscopic examination of those tumors showed, however, that they were composed of the same eight to fourteen well-differentiated cell types that were present in the original tumor together with embryonal carcinoma cells.

Differentiated cell types present in the tumor were found, moreover, to have lost their tumorous properties. Since all of the cells present in these teratocarcinomas were derived from the single cancer cells that were injected into mice and since differentiated cell types present in those tumors had lost their malignant properties, it must be concluded that as the embryonal carcinoma cells divide they regularly give rise to cells that are nontumorous. The results of this study clearly demonstrate, then, that the embryonal carcinoma cell is a multipotential cell which is highly malignant in the undifferentiated state but is capable of giving rise to a broad spectrum of differentiated cell types that have lost their malignant properties. Studies on this tumor have now been carried one additional step and the reported results are truly remarkable. Instead of implanting a single cancer cell into a whole mouse as was done in the experiments described above, a single embryonal carcinoma cell was injected into a very young mouse embryo before the normal cells present in the embryo had yet been determined as to the precise cell types into which those cells would ultimately differentiate (122). Specific markers were available which allowed the investigators to follow the fate of the progeny of the single cancer cell during the development of the embryo into a mature mouse. The results of this study showed that the mosaic mice that developed in these studies were composed of both normal cells and cells derived from the implanted cancer cell. The cancer-derived cells were found, moreover, to make a very substantial contribution to all of a wide range of tissues and organs found in the adult mosaic mice and those cancer-derived cells therefore differentiated into numerous normal directions including the production of functional liver, kidney, and thymus gland cells as well as reproductively functional sperm, none of which are found in the teratocarcinoma itself. Certain of the adult mosaic mice were found to be free of cancer despite the fact that their tissues and organs were composed in significant part of cancer-derived cells. The results of this study provide additional yet very dramatic evidence that those morphogenetic factors and regulatory mechanisms that govern so precisely growth, cellular differentiation, as well as tissue and organ formation during the normal course of development can remodel the metabolic patterns present in a cancer cell in such a way that perfectly normal patterns of growth, cellular differentiation, and function occur. The fact, moreover, that the cancer-derived cells participated in the development of most and perhaps all of the specialized cell types found in a normal adult mouse indicates that such cells are totipotential and therefore have retained while in the cancerous state all of the genetic information necessary to, potentially at least, reconstitute an entirely normal mouse.

## Squamous Cell Carcinoma of the Rat

The partial and even the complete self-healing of cancer cells present in the teratocarcinoma of the mouse is, then, a characteristic feature of that tumor. There are other cancers of mammals and man that behave similarly. One of the more commonly found examples of this is the epidermoid (squamous) carcinoma. This type of tumor may be readily initiated in an experimental animal such as the rat by ionizing radiation. This cancer originates from the basal cells of the skin or of the hair follicles. It is well known that when a normal basal cell divides it gives rise to one cell that differentiates, becomes keratinized, and forms the outer layer of the skin while the other member of the divided pair retains the properties of and replaces the basal cell from which it was derived. The epidermoid (squamous) carcinoma typically consists of an agglomeration of epidermal cell pegs which are embedded in a matrix of normal connective tissue (see Fig. 22). When such tumor pegs are examined under a microscope it can be seen that only the cancer cells that are found at the rim of each peg grow and divide actively

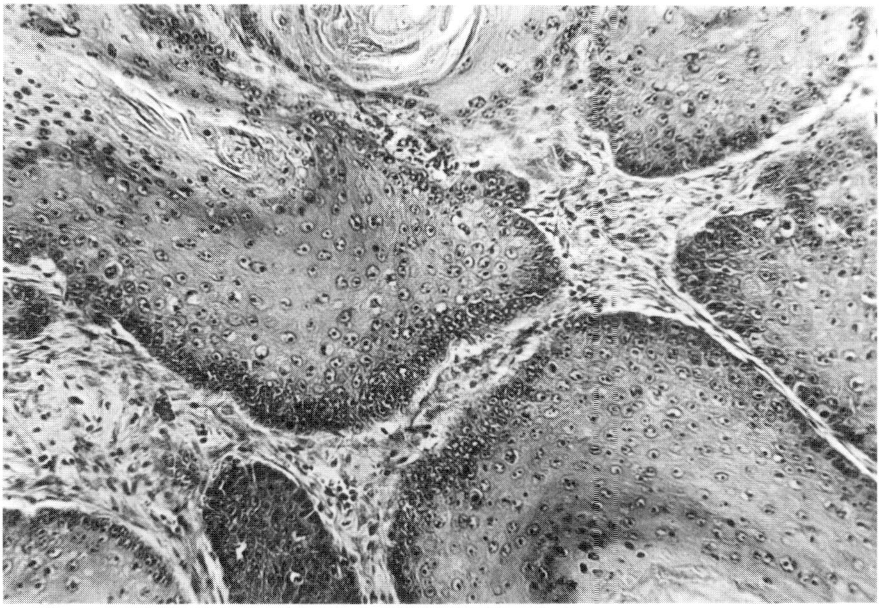

FIGURE 22. Histological section of an epidermoid (squamous) carcinoma of the rat that was induced by ionizing radiation. Structurally this tumor consists of an agglomeration of epidermal cell pegs which are embedded in a matrix of normal connective tissue. Cell division occurs in the cancer cells that are found at the rim of each peg while the centers of the pegs are composed of heavily keratinized cells that no longer appear capable of division. The differentiated cells at the center of the pegs, although derived from the actively dividing cancer cells at the rim of the pegs, are terminally differentiated and have lost their cancerous properties. (Courtesy of Dr. Roy E. Albert)

while the cells at the inside of a peg have become differentiated, contain large amounts of keratin, and no longer divide. A study was undertaken to determine the origin of the differentiated cells at the center of the pegs and it was found that they were derived from the dividing cancer cells at the outer rim of the peg (123). It was reported further that when the actively dividing cancer cells were isolated from the tumor and implanted into appropriate hosts they developed into typical epidermoid (squamous) carcinomas. When, on the other hand, the cancer-derived differentiated cells present in the centers of the pegs were similarly implanted into appropriate animals, tumors did not develop. It thus appears that the cancer cell is behaving like a normal basal cell in that when it divides it gives rise to one cell that differentiates and, in this instance, loses its cancerous properties while the other member of the divided pair retains its cancerous properties. Here, then, is another example of a cancer in mammals including humans the cells of which characteristically retain their potentialities for differentiation with the loss of their cancerous properties. It is clear, moreover, that all of the genetic information necessary for the development of a specific type of differentiation must have been retained by the malignant cells since a large part of such tumors is composed of cancer cells that have differentiated into nontumorous skin cells. It is evident, furthermore, that all the cells of such cancers retain the potentialities to differentiate into nontumorous cell types, and the problem of control of such cancers would appear to resolve itself into learning how to bring about the controlled expression of those potentialities in all cells of such tumors.

## Lucké Adenocarcinoma of the Frog

Are there, then, experimental test systems available which could provide a clue to the nature of the cellular mechanisms and substances that are responsible for reprogramming the genetic information present in a cancer cell nucleus in such a way that it leads again to the normal phenotype? A cancerous disease of the common leopard frog which is known as the Lucké adenocarcinoma appears admirably suited for such studies. This highly malignant tumor is caused by a specific virus (a herpes-type virus) and is commonly found to occur in frogs in the New England States. The virus in this instance rather specifically transforms certain kidney cells, the convoluted tubules, into cancer cells. It was indicated earlier in this discussion that when nuclei such as those found in normal differentiated intestinal epithelial cells of the African clawed toad are implanted into activated normal toad eggs from which the normal nucleus of the egg had been removed, the nuclei from the specialized epithelial cells served to direct development along normal pathways and completely normal toads developed. Those specialized normal cell nuclei were therefore totipotential since the progeny of those nuclei were capable of reconstituting an entirely normal organism. It was of interest to learn, therefore, what would happen if a nucleus from a Lucké cancer cell was implanted into an activated normal frog egg from which the normal nucleus had been removed. This experiment has now been done and most remarkable results have been reported (124). The cancer nucleus behaved like a normal nucleus in that it directed perfectly normal development to proceed to the tadpole stage (see Fig. 23). In these studies fully functional tadpoles, which contained all of the specialized cell types, tissues, and organs present in normal tadpoles of comparable age and stage of development, were obtained. Despite the fact that each of these tadpoles was derived from a cancer nucleus there was no evidence of cancer in them. The results of this study illustrate very dramatically that the genetic information present in a cancer nucleus need not be irreversibly fixed, as was believed for so many years, but that it can, in fact, be reprogramed in such a way as to permit normal development to proceed at least to the tadpole stage. Those cytoplasmic factors and mechanisms present in a normal frog egg that influence the expression of the genetic information present in a normal frog nucleus can also influence the expression of the genetic information present in a

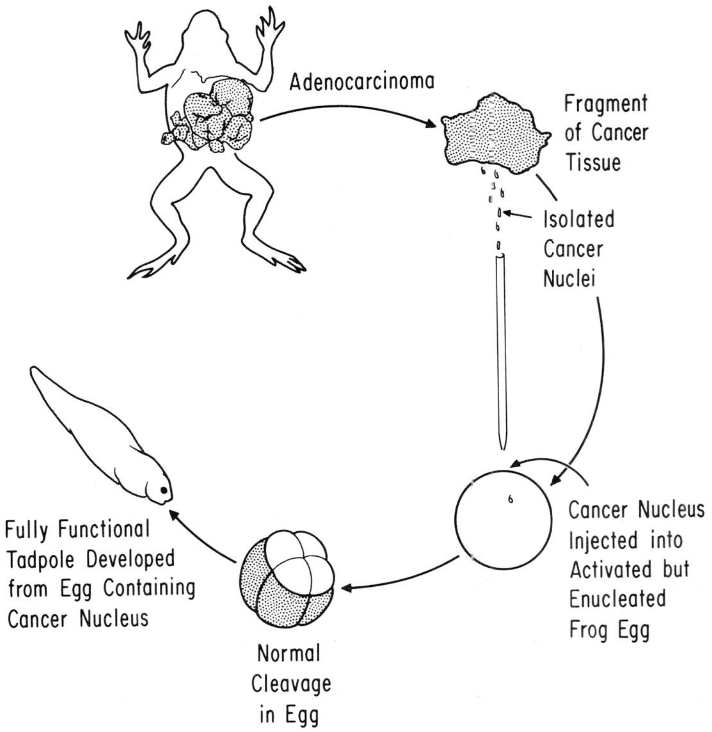


FIGURE 23. The results of this study illustrate the developmental potentialities of a cancer nucleus derived from a Lucké adenocarcinoma cell. When such a cancer nucleus is isolated and implanted into an activated but enucleated normal frog egg cleavage occurs and apparently normal, fully functional tadpoles develop. The results of this study provide evidence to show that the cytoplasmic factors and regulatory mechanisms present in a normal frog egg can reprogram the genetic information present in a cancer nucleus in such a way as to permit normal development to proceed to the tadpole stage.

cancer nucleus in such a way that the cancer nucleus behaves in effect as does a normal nucleus. An understanding of the nature of the cytoplasmic factors and mechanisms that are present in a normal egg cell and that can so profoundly influence gene expression in both normal and cancer nuclei would appear most important to an understanding of the biology of the cancer problem. The results of this study show us, moreover, that the genetic information present in the Lucké cancer nucleus has been conserved sufficiently to permit perfectly normal development to proceed at least as far as the tadpole stage.

Cells of the Lucké adenocarcinoma, like most cancer cells, appear by generally accepted criteria to be irreversibly altered cells. Yet, the nuclear transplantation studies described above indicate that that is not necessarily true. It was only because of the truly unique characteristics of the experimental test system used in that study, as well as in other studies reported above, that the possibility of reprograming the genetic information present in a tumor cell nucleus could be approached in so direct a manner with so definitive an answer.

Some of the more practical minded might well ask what all of this has to do with cancer as a clinical problem. A search of the literature shows numerous examples in which a partial or, very occasionally, a complete self-healing of advanced cancers of man occurs spontaneously. Some of the best documented examples of this are found in the neuroblastomas of man.

## The Neuroblastomas of Humans

The neuroblastoma is a highly malignant cancer of humans that is derived from immature nerve cells, the neuroblasts. This disease is commonly found in infants, it spreads rapidly through the body, and in the vast majority of patients there is a rapid downhill course culminating in death in a relatively few months. There are now a significant number of dramatic and well documented exceptions to this in which all of the cells of advanced metastasizing neuroblastomas matured and differentiated spontaneously into ganglion cells that had lost their cancerous properties (125-128). Patients in whom such spontaneous regressions occurred lived for many years without recurrence of the malignant tumor. If this sort of thing can occur spontaneously in the human body there clearly must be an underlying cause, and the problem of control in this instance would depend upon a precise characterization of that cause.

## SPECIFIC SUBSTANCES INVOLVED IN THE REVERSION OF TUMOR CELLS TO NORMAL CELLS

Attempts have now been made to cause neuroblastoma cells to differentiate into mature nerve cells by applying specific substances to those cells under conditions of cell culture. The first of these substances is the nerve growth factor which has been found to be importantly involved in causing normal immature nerve cells to differentiate into mature nerve cells. When this substance is applied to neuroblastoma cells in culture it also causes those cells to mature into ganglion-like cells, thus indicating that the cancer cells retain, in this instance, the potentialities for differentiation into more mature cell types. A second substance that has been found to influence the maturation of neuroblastoma cells is a non-naturally occurring substance known as dimethylsulfoxide (see Fig. 24). When this substance was applied to neuroblastoma cells it also caused those cells to mature into ganglion-like cells which remained in a stable, nondividing state for periods up to one month and acquired a high degree of electrical excitability which is characteristic of normal nerve cells (129). Dimethylsulfoxide had earlier been shown by others to cause cells of an erythroleukemia (leukemia that originates in a red blood cell line) of the mouse to mature,

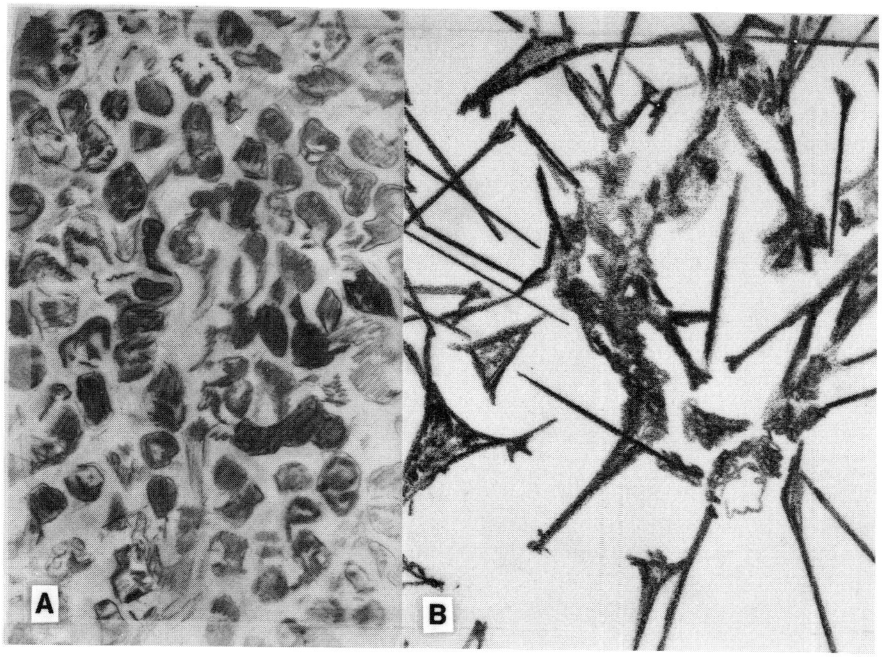


FIGURE 24. Drawings of (A) neuroblastoma cells as they commonly appear in a host and (B) when they are isolated and treated with dimethylsulfoxide in culture.

differentiate, and behave for the time being in every respect as if they were normal cells (130).

A naturally occurring, essentially nontoxic substance has also been found to profoundly influence the growth and differentiation of acute leukemic cells of humans. This substance has variously come to be known as the MGI protein (131), the colony stimulating factor or the colony stimulating activity (132, 133). This substance removes the block for differentiation that is present in acute myelogenous leukemic cells of humans. This differentiation-inducing protein is released in culture by a number of normal cell types and when applied to the leukemic cells causes those cells to mature and differentiate into two types of normal white blood cells, the granulocytes and macrophages, which have lost their cancerous properties. Because of the essentially nontoxic nature of this substance and because of its specific effects on inducing differentiation in leukemic cells, it has been suggested that this substance may be of potential value for the treatment of acute leukemia in humans (131).

Some progress appears now to have been made in an attempt to characterize cellular factors and mechanisms that lead to terminal differentiation of tumor cells in higher plant species. It is a common observation that plant tumors of many different kinds growing not only in a host but as cloned lines in culture contain terminally differentiated cells that are known as tracheary elements (see Fig. 25). The differentiation of tumor cells into tracheary elements represents an attempt by the tumor to vascularize since tracheary elements are components of the normal vascular (xylem) system of plants. The potentialities for this type of cytodifferentiation are clearly present in cells of many different plant tumors. Since this represents a form of terminal differentiation with a loss of tumorous properties, it seemed reasonable to assume

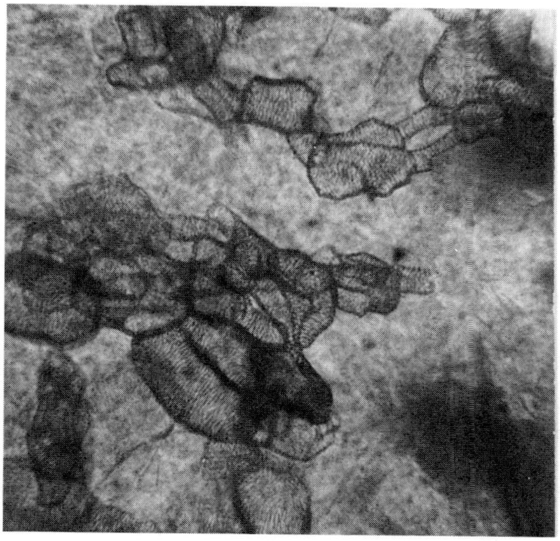

FIGURE 25. Tracheary elements of the type that differentiate spontaneously from plant tumor cells of many different kinds. These tracheary elements are highly lignified, terminally differentiated cells that have lost their tumorous properties. Compare with the epidermoid (squamous) carcinoma of the rat shown in Figure 22 in which the derivatives of the cancer cells have become heavily keratinized and terminally differentiated with a loss of their tumorous properties.

that if the inductive and other factors underlying this type of cytodifferentiation were fully understood, it might be possible to reprogram the genetic information present in all cells of such tumors and thus effect a recovery from the tumorous state. The results of that study have shown that the regulation of cyclic AMP(3'5') (or the higher plant equivalent of that substance) is somehow importantly involved in inducing the formation of tracheary elements (134). While the readily degradable, naturally occurring cyclic AMP(3'5') was ineffective in inducing tracheary element formation, the highly stable 8-bromo derivative of that compound was found to be highly effective. The available evidence suggests that the 8-bromo derivative of cAMP(3'5') may be exerting its biological effects by virtue of the fact that it is a structural analog of the naturally occurring cAMP(3'5') and is competing with that compound for active sites on the phosphodiesterase enzymes which, in turn, are importantly involved in regulating the levels of the naturally occurring cyclic nucleotide in cells. Certain other known phosphodiesterase inhibitors (theophylline and cytokinesin I) have been found to be effective in inducing the formation of tracheary elements in cells of higher plant species. The 8-bromo derivative of cAMP(3'5') has now also been shown to encourage the differentiation of undetermined presumptive epidermis into simple "motor neurons" and "central nervous system neurons" in certain amphibians (135).

The studies reported above clearly demonstrate that it is possible, in certain select instances at least, to manipulate nuclear gene function in a tumor cell in such a way as to cause it to revert to the normal phenotype. Before concluding this section we might reasonably raise the question why, if tumor cells contain a complete complement of genes, are not all tumor cells totipotent and thus capable of giving rise under appropriate conditions to all cell types found in an organism. Why, in other words, are the progeny of single tumor cells of tobacco or single teratocarcinoma cells of the mouse able to differentiate into all of the diverse specialized cell types found in their respective hosts, while the tumor cells of the epidermoid (squamous) carcinoma differentiate only into special types of skin cells and cells of the neuroblastoma differentiate only into nerve cells? The plant teratoma cells and the teratocarcinoma cells of the mouse retain their broad potentialities for differentiation because they have not been determined for differentiation in a specific direction at the time of their transformation while the basal cell of the skin, from which the epidermoid carcinoma arises, or the immature nerve cell, which gives rise to neuroblastoma cells, are specifically determined for the cell types into which they are destined to differentiate. Thus, although cells of the latter two tumors may contain a complete complement of genes, those genes are specifically programed for particular patterns of differentiation that are not easily manipulated experimentally.

It should perhaps also be mentioned here that a recovery from the tumorous state does not necessarily mean a reversion to the normal state. As will be pointed out later in this discussion, many secondary changes (abnormal chromosome numbers, alteration in respiration, deletion of enzymatic activities, etc.) may and commonly do occur in certain tumors. Thus, even if those cellular properties that lead to the tumorous state were potentially reversible the result would not necessarily be a normal cell since the recovered cell might retain the secondarily acquired properties possessed by the tumor cell. Even though such a reverted cell would be abnormal it would, nevertheless, be nontumorous and thus fulfill the criteria for reversion from the tumorous to the nontumorous state.

The results of all of these studies demonstrate, then, that the tumorous state present in cells found in a wide spectrum of tumors that range in origin from those found in higher plant species to select tumors that occur in frogs, mice, rats, as well as in certain cancers found in humans, is reversible, leading to a normalization of the tumorous state. The implication of this is that all of the genetic information necessary to establish and maintain the tumorous state is present in normal cells, is retained but is expressed differently when those cells are converted into tumor cells, and is again expressed in the original way when the tumor cells revert to the normal state. These studies provide very strong experimental evidence to indicate that whether the normal phenotype or tumor phenotype is expressed depends upon the persistent activation or repression of specific genes present in the total genetic information found in a cell. If that is true, then the basic cellular mechanisms that underlie the tumorous state are similar to those that underlie cellular differentiation that occurs during the normal course of development of an organism. The tumor problem would then simply be a problem of anomalous differentiation and its expression would be subject to many of the same regulatory mechanisms that govern normal growth and development in an organism. This matter will be considered further in Chapter VII.

# CHAPTER V

# NATURE OF THE HERITABLE CELLULAR CHANGE, II. SOMATIC MUTATION

The demonstration that the tumorous state can arise and be perpetuated in the presence of a complete and unaltered complement of host cell genes permits us to conclude that drastic changes of a mutational type involving the deletion or permanent rearrangement of the genetic information present in a cell are not an essential prerequisite for either the establishment or for the maintenance of the tumorous state. This does not, of course, necessarily mean that heritable changes of a mutational nature could not be involved and the mutation theory has in the past and continues to appeal to many as a likely mechanism for the origin of many cancers. This theory as a heritable cellular mechanism underlying tumorigenesis has over the years engendered controversy which often was based more on emotional responses or on personal whims than on hard experimental evidence. The American pathologist and Nobel Laureate Peyton Rous wrote in 1959 that there is little evidence for the somatic mutation hypothesis and that the introduction of that theory into the cancer literature has resulted in "no good thing but much that is bad." He continued that it has led to "fatalism to blast many a hope and effort." Yet in discussing this matter Rous offered no viable alternative (136). Some of the more ardent proponents of the mutation theory have, on the other hand, often regarded that theory as being so obviously true that its validity should perhaps not even be questioned. Because the nature of the heritable cellular change that underlies the tumorous state represents one of the major pieces of our cancer jigsaw puzzle, it would appear necessary to critically analyze this question and attempt to determine the validity of the mutation theory as it applies to the tumor problem. One of the difficulties in discussing mutation as a mechanism underlying the tumorous state is that definitions often used by proponents of that theory are so vague as to be essentially meaningless as a basis for discussion. For example, the author of a book dealing with the origin of cancer has stated: "the premises justifying the conclusion that mutation takes place begins [sic] with dicta on biological behaviour that have been accepted for a century or more. If 'all cells come from pre-existing cells,' as proclaimed by Virchow in 1855; and 'all cells come from genetically similar parent cells,' as asserted by Thiersch 10 years later; and cancer cells originate from normal body cells, then somewhere along the line of change from normalcy to malignancy there must be one or more mutations" (137). Reasoning such as this is not at all uncommon and clearly precludes the existence of heritable cellular changes other than those caused by mutations at the nuclear gene level.

If the term somatic mutation is used, as it often is, to describe the obvious fact that a profound and heritable change occurs during the conversion of a normal cell to a tumor cell, then it is pretentious as a descriptive term and carries with it a connotation that tends to stifle precision of thought. If, on the other hand, by somatic mutation is meant that there is a permanent alteration in the genetic determinants present in the nucleus of a cell, then the term designates an hypothesis that remains untestable by classical Mendelian methods because tumor cells propagate themselves only by cell divisions and cannot therefore be subjected to Mendelian analysis. The newer method of somatic cell hybridization, which we will consider later in this discussion, may ultimately assist in clarifying this matter.

There are good, although not in themselves sufficient, reasons why the mutation hypothesis as it applies to the tumor problem has had such a strong appeal over the years for cancer biologists and these may be listed as follows. The fact that the characteristic properties of tumor cells, like genetic traits generally, are transmitted to their progeny over long periods of time and since these newly acquired traits are abnormal and often appear irreversible, it has been assumed that something drastic, such as a mutation(s), must have occurred in the genetic material present in a tumor cell. It is also true that radiation and the carcinogenic chemicals are not only powerful cancer-producing agents but are also effective in causing mutations. The fact, moreover, that the wavelengths of ultraviolet light that are effective in inducing tumors are those that are preferentially absorbed by and that damage the structure of the nucleic acids, suggests that an etiological relationship exists. Certain of the cancer-producing chemicals are known, moreover, to react chemically with the nucleic acids and proteins in a cell. Finally, cells treated with either physical or chemical carcinogens, whether they are converted to the tumorous state or not, often show abnormal chromosome numbers as well as breaks in the chromosomes. Such chromosomal abnormalities are also found in many advanced tumors growing in an organism. It is also true that in certain instances in which a specific mutation is known to exist in all cells of an organism, as for example in a rare human disease known as retinoblastoma or where cells of an individual contain an abnormal number of chromosomes as in the case of patients with Fanconia's anemia or Down's syndrome, proneness for the development of tumors including cancers is heightened appreciably. All of these findings would appear to provide powerful support for the mutation theory for the origin of cancer and yet in few, if any, instances has a causal relationship been unequivocally established. It might be profitable, therefore, to examine briefly each of the points raised above to see if acceptable alternatives to the mutation theory can be suggested.

## ABNORMAL CHROMOSOMES IN TUMOR CELLS

It is, of course, well known that abnormal numbers of chromosomes are found in cells of many advanced tumors and it is often possible to find that different cells within a given tumor contain variable but abnormal numbers of chromosomes. It is, nevertheless, also true that a number of cancers have now been found the cells of which contain a normal complement of chromosomes, indicating that abnormal numbers of chromosomes need not necessarily be involved (138-140). The fact, moreover, that the cells of many early tumors contain a normal complement of chromosomes has led to the suggestion that deviations from the original diploid complement of chromosomes found in advanced tumors may be regarded as manifestations of genetic evolution in which the dominant cell line represents those cells that contain chromosome numbers that are best adapted to their immediate environment (141). Thus, cells with different numbers of chromosomes within a given tumor could confer a very real selective advantage as far as growth of the tumor is concerned.

While the generality of advanced cancers do not show characteristic abnormal chromosome numbers there are certain exceptions to this. One of these is found in chronic myelocytic leukemia of humans. A correlation has been found to exist in this instance between the presence of an abnormal chromosome and the disease. The so-called Philadelphia chromosome ($Ph^1$), which is chromosome number 22 in the human cell, has, in this instance, lost approximately one-half of its long arm and this chromosome defect is believed to be a specific morphological marker for this disease (142). Recent studies suggest that the chromosome part is not lost from the cell but is translocated from the Philadelphia chromosome to chromosome 9 and is replicated with that chromosome (143). This, then, would appear to be a classic example of a somatic mutation involving the permanent rearrangement of some of the genetic information present in the tumor cell. Yet it is difficult to know what the correlation that has been found to exist between the $Ph^1$ chromosome and the disease means because the correlation is not a perfect one since it has been found to exist in only 85 to 90 percent of typical cases of chronic myelocytic leukemia studied (142). The remaining 10 to 15 percent of the cases appear to show an essentially normal chromosome picture, which would suggest that the presence of the $Ph^1$ chromosome is not an essential prerequisite for the development of the disease. The fact, moreover, that the $Ph^1$ chromosome has been found to be present in granulocytic cells of a few individuals who did not develop the disease indicates that the presence of that chromosome is not in itself sufficient to cause the disease. It may well be, therefore, that the presence of the $Ph^1$ chromosome renders those cells particularly vulnerable to some environmental cancer-producing agent rather than itself being specifically involved in establishing and maintaining the disease.

There are, as indicated above, certain rather rare diseases (Fanconia's anemia and Down's syndrome), in which the cells of an afflicted individual contain an abnormal complement of chromosomes and proneness for the development of cancers in these individuals is increased significantly.

What, if anything, the abnormal chromosome picture has to do with the increased incidence of cancer in these instances is not known since in both of these diseases there is found a marked insufficiency of the immune response which could in itself explain the higher incidence of cancer found in those individuals. It has also been reported that cells of patients with Fanconia's anemia are far more susceptible to transformation with certain cancer-producing viruses (SV40) than are comparable normal human cells (144). All of this does not, of course, mean that tumors cannot arise as the result of chromosomal imbalance and this theory, which is favored in some quarters at the present time, will now be illustrated with the use of select examples.

It has been found that cells of hamsters that have been transformed to the tumorous state by oncogenic viruses (145), chemical carcinogens (72), or by X-irradiation (71), can revert to cells that appear normal. This reversion from the tumorous state to the "normal" state can be induced with high frequency when the tumor cells are plated in culture in low cell density (146). The normal hamster cells contain 44 chromosomes. It was found, however, that the cells that had reverted from tumor to "normal" did not contain the typical complement of chromosomes but instead contained either somewhat more (147) or somewhat less (148) than the normal 44 chromosomes. On the basis of these studies it was suggested that malignancy and its reversion to the "normal" state is controlled by a balance between genes for expression and genes for suppression of the tumorous state (147). Thus, when genes for tumor suppression predominate, malignancy is suppressed; while when genes for tumor expression dominate, the malignant phenotype is expressed, a situation that could well result from chromosomal imbalance in cells. Recent studies suggest that changes in chromosome numbers need not accompany the reversion of a tumor cell to a "normal" cell. Using other experimental test systems, it was reported that an abnormal karyotype is not essential for the reversion to "normal" (149). Other types of experiments have demonstrated that when certain essentially normal cells were allowed to fuse in culture with several different kinds of malignant cells, the cancerous state in the progeny of the hybrid cell was largely suppressed and those cells behaved in a normal manner (150, 151). That the suppression of the malignant state was due to some contribution made by the genes present on chromosomes of the normal cell line is evidenced by the fact that this contribution is lost and the cells again become fully malignant when certain chromosomes of the normal cell line are eliminated from the progeny of the hybrid cells. The factor(s) responsible for the suppression of malignancy thus has its origin on one or more of the chromosomes of the normal cell line. This could mean either that certain of the normal chromosomes are coding for some tumor-suppressing factor or that the cytoplasmic environment created by the presence of the normal chromosomes is temporarily reprograming the genetic information present on the tumor chromosomes so that they are not producing tumor-promoting factors.

## INTERSPECIFIC HYBRIDS AND TUMORS

It has also been found that when crosses are made between related species of animals or plants the resulting hybrids may develop tumors spontaneously and in large numbers. When, for example, backcrosses are made from the $F_1$ hybrids of two species of fish, the swordtail and the platyfish, melanomas develop in these hybrids which may expand rapidly and may be fatal (152). Similarly, when the wild gray mouse is crossed with an inbred strain of the domestic mouse the incidence of tumors in the hybrids has been found to be tenfold higher than is the sum of the parental incidence (153). Particularly well analyzed examples of this are found in plants in the case of certain interspecific hybrids within the genus *Nicotiana* (tobacco) (70) (see Fig. 26). When two plant species such as *Nicotiana glauca* which has 24 chromosomes in its

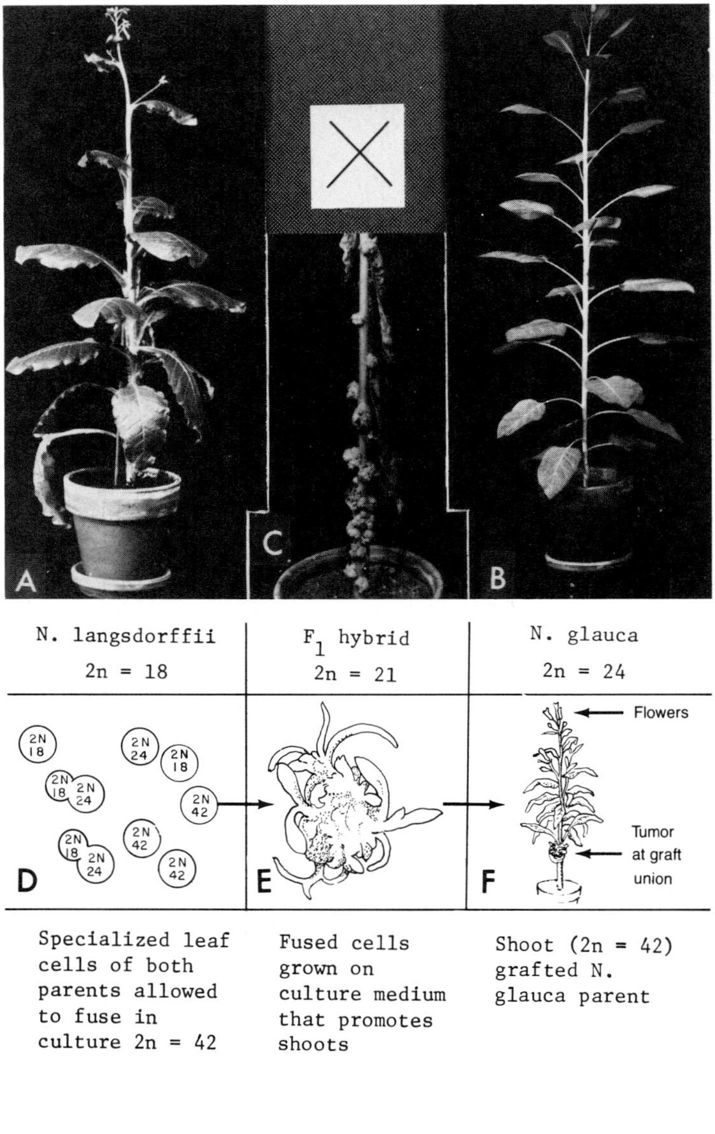


FIGURE 26. This figure illustrates the Kostoff genetic tumors of plants. When (A) Nicotiana langsdorffii (2n = 18) is crossed with (B) Nicotiana glauca (2n = 24) the resulting $F_1$ hybrid (2n = 21) (C) invariably develops tumors spontaneously on all parts of the plant. The hybrid plant flowers but does not set viable seed. If specialized leaf (mesophyll) cells are isolated from the two parental species (A) and (B)

cells (2n = 24) and Nicotiana langsdorffii which has 18 chromosomes (2n = 18) are crossed and the seed of the hybrid which has 21 chromosomes (2n = 21) are sown, the resulting plants commonly grow normally until they reach maturity at which time a profusion of tumors invariably arise spontaneously from all parts of such plants. It has been found that when specialized cell types are isolated from leaves of both parent species and grown separately in culture and then mixed together to permit fusion of cells from the two parents to occur, the resulting hybrid cells contained, as would be expected, 42 chromosomes. These hybrid cells were isolated and grown separately in culture under conditions that favored the development of shoots. When such shoots were grafted to appropriate stock plants they grew in an organized manner and some of these not only flowered and set fertile seed but spontaneous tumors often developed at the point at which the shoot was grafted to the stock plant (154). This experimental

and allowed to fuse in culture (D) the resulting hybrid cells contain 42 chromosomes. When these cells are grown on an inductive medium they organize shoots (E). When such shoots are grafted to the N. glauca parent they may not only develop in an apparently normal manner and flower and set viable seed but they commonly produce tumors spontaneously at the graft union (F). Thus, the same abnormal complement of chromosomes in all cells of the hybrid plant can give rise, on the one hand, to tumorous growths and, on the other, to normal-appearing plants that set viable seed.

test system appears to be particularly illuminating because it clearly demonstrates that despite serious chromosomal imbalance in all cells of the hybrid plant, the same abnormal complement of chromosomes can give rise, on the one hand, to normal-appearing plants that flower and set viable seed, indicating that all of the genetic information necessary to reconstitute a plant is present in those cells. That same abnormal chromosome complement can, on the other hand, give rise spontaneously to tumorous growths. These two metastable states are readily reversible in both directions. These findings provide excellent evidence in support of the concept that the tumorous state, like normal developmental processes, may stem from persistent changes in the expression of a genetically equivalent, although in this instance abnormal, chromosome complement in all cells of the plant.

## MECHANISMS OTHER THAN MUTATIONS INVOLVED IN TUMORIGENESIS

It is, of course, possible that very small changes in the integrity of the genetic information present in a cell occur and that it is those changes rather than gross changes such as those associated with abnormal chromosome numbers that are involved in establishing the tumorous state. It has been found, for example, that when certain cells such as hamster cells are converted into tumor cells by a virus--in this instance the Rous sarcoma virus--breaks occur in the chromosomes and such breaks may involve specific chromosomes more often than others. It has been suggested that such chromosome breaks may be significant and may act as an indicator system for point mutations (155). Subsequent studies showed, however, that when a reversion from the tumorous state to the "normal" state occurred, this resulted from the fact that the viral genetic information present in the reverted cell had become suppressed (156). It thus appears that the observed breaks in the chromosomes could not have been involved in establishing the tumorous state. Whether the viral genetic information is turned on or off in a cell rather than mutations resulting from chromosome breaks appears in this instance to determine the fate of the cell.

There are certain tumors that arise in individuals all of whose cells are known to contain mutations. One of the more interesting of these is a tumorous disease of the eye in humans that is known as retinoblastoma. This disease is inherited as a recessive trait and appears in children who have inherited a single recessive mutant gene from each parent. The presence of these recessive genes would not appear to be the cause of the cancer because the mutant genes are present in all cells of such an individual and one finds that such tumors arise only in specific cells of the eyes. While these tumors often arise in both of the eyes at about the same time, many instances have been reported in which a tumor develops in only one of the eyes. This is true despite the fact that the mutant genes are present in the retinal cells of both of the eyes and those cells proceed through precisely the same developmental stages until the time that the tumor is initiated. It would thus appear that the mutant genes are not the immediate cause of retinoblastoma since the presence of those genes is not in itself sufficient to cause a tumor to be initiated. The mutant genes must, nevertheless, play an important role in predisposing certain specific cells of the eye to the tumorous conversion either by rendering such cells particularly vulnerable to a persistent misprograming of genetic information during a specific stage in their differentiation, by making certain retinal cells unusually susceptible to some cancer-producing agent, or possibly, as has been suggested, that one or more additional mutations occur which render the cells tumorous (157).

One of the most appealing arguments advanced by proponents of the mutation theory of cancer is the presumed correlation that exists between the capacity of an agent to cause mutations in the genetic material present in a cell and its ability to convert normal cells into tumor cells.

Radiation and cancer-producing chemicals are often not only powerful cancer-inducing agents but are potent mutagens as well. Does this, then, necessarily mean, as is often implied, that since those agents may cause mutations it is those mutations that are responsible for the establishment and maintenance of the tumorous state?

It is now well known that radiation can cause tumors by at least two and possibly a third mechanism other than that postulated for somatic mutation at the nuclear gene level. It was believed for many years that certain leukemias that arose in mice following exposure of the mice to X-irradiation were the result of somatic mutations. It has been found, however, that these leukemias are caused by specific viruses which are present in cells of mice in a latent or inactive form (158, 159). Following irradiation, those viruses become oncologically active and cause the cancers to develop. When those viruses are isolated from the leukemic cells and allowed to infect appropriate normal non-irradiated cells they regularly transform those cells into tumor cells. Thus X-irradiation, in these instances, is clearly not inducing the tumorous state by virtue of the fact that it acts by causing mutations at the nuclear gene level.

A second and quite different example of tumors that result from radiation and are not due to mutations are those that arise in the ovaries of mice following exposure of the animals to radiation (160). The development of two types of ovarian tumors which are known as luteomas and granulosa cell tumors can be prevented by shielding one of the ovaries from the source of radiation or by injecting the female sex hormone estrogen into the irradiated animals. The results of these studies suggest, then, that tumors arose in the irradiated ovaries because of a reduced production of estrogen. This reduced production of estrogen led, in turn, to an increased production of another hormone, known as gonadotrophin, which is produced by the pituitary gland. When this increase in gonadotrophin was prevented, tumors did not develop in the ovaries despite the fact that they had been exposed to the same dose of radiation that commonly led to the development of the tumors. It seems clear that in this instance tumors arise as the result of disturbances in growth regulatory mechanisms rather than from somatic mutations at the nuclear gene level.

It was indicated earlier in this discussion that prolonged exposure to strong sunlight and particularly to the ultraviolet region of the spectrum can lead to the development of certain cancers of the skin. This finding was widely interpreted to mean that the ultraviolet light damages the genetic material present in a cell. Yet it has recently been found that when cells of human skin or those of hairless skin of mice are exposed to ultraviolet light a compound with known cancer-producing properties, cholesterol-α-oxide, is produced in the skin cells (26). The finding that normal skin cholesterol can be converted into a cancer-producing chemical in the presence of ultraviolet light provides a possible alternative mechanism to that postulating damage to the genetic information present in a cell as the cause of the tumorous state. There is, nevertheless, a rather rare disease of humans known as xeroderma pigmentosum in which tumors appear to be genetically determined. This disease is due to a recessive gene and occurs in individuals who have inherited this recessive gene from both parents. Such individuals, however, develop cancers only if they are exposed to strong sunlight or other forms of radiation. What is obviously transmitted in this instance is not the cancer but rather the two recessive genes which then predispose the skin exposed to strong sunlight to the development of cancer. Recent studies have shown that although irradiation with ultraviolet light damages the nucleic acids equally in normal human skin cells and in cells from individuals with xeroderma pigmentosum, the resulting damage is quickly repaired in the normal cells while damage in the case of xeroderma pigmentosum skin is not (161). It was suggested that an inability to repair the damaged DNA may be the cause of tumor formation in this instance.

## RELATIONSHIP BETWEEN MUTAGENICITY AND CARCINOGENICITY IN BACTERIA

Methods designed to screen potential cancer-producing chemicals rapidly and cheaply are, of course, most desirable. One of the methods that has attracted considerable interest recently makes use of mutant strains of a specific bacterium, *Salmonella typhimurium*. It has been claimed that a high correlation exists between the ability of compounds to cause specific types of mutations (frameshift mutations and/or base-pair substitutions) in the bacteria and the cancer-producing ability of the tested compounds in mammals. It has been suggested, further, that since the cancer-producing substances cause mutations in the bacteria, they cause cancers in mammalian cells by the same mechanisms (162). An analysis of the data that has thus far been presented suggests, however, that caution must be exercised for a number of reasons before arriving at that conclusion (163, 164).

Whether potential cancer-producing substances cause mutations of the frameshift type in bacteria is commonly determined in the following manner. A nutritionally deficient mutant strain of a bacterium that does not grow in a particular culture medium is treated with a substance to be tested for its potential cancer-producing effects, usually in the presence of enzymes that convert many carcinogens into their ultimate active forms. The bacteria do not produce those enzymes. Following treatment, the bacteria are plated in the culture medium and if colonies now develop it is taken as evidence that a frameshift mutation has occurred and, by inference, that the substance is cancer-producing by the same mechanism in cells of animals and humans. In other words, a cancer-producing substance is believed to repair the damage in the nutritionally deficient test strain of the bacteria while non-cancer-producing substances are presumed not to be effective in that respect. It has been reported (162) that such well known and potent carcinogens as, for example, methylcholanthrene and 2-aminoanthracene produce under the best conditions 510 and 11,200 frameshift mutations, respectively, at a particular gene locus (the histidine locus) for every 200 to 300 million bacterial cells treated with those substances. Great differences have, however, been found to exist in the sensitivity to develop frameshift mutations in different mutant strains of bacteria having a defect at the same genetic locus. For example, when the histidine-deficient mutant strain TA1535 of <u>Salmonella typhimurium</u> was treated with methylcholanthrene, 22 revertant colonies were obtained as compared with 11 colonies in the controls that did not contain the carcinogen; while when strain TA1358 was used and similarly treated, 510 revertant colonies developed as compared with 46 in the controls. Thus, if tested against strain TA1535, methylcholanthrene would be considered marginal at best in its ability to produce frameshift mutations and, by implication, to act as a carcinogen in humans, and yet we know it to be a very potent cancer-producing agent when applied to animals. That strain TA1535 is capable of developing mutations of the frameshift type at the same histidine-defective locus is evidenced by the fact that 318 revertant colonies were obtained when the bacterial cells were treated with another known carcinogen, 2-aminoanthracene, as compared in this instance with 16 revertants in the controls. It has thus been pointed out, and perhaps correctly, that the bacterial strains used to test mutagenicity were obtained through genetic manipulation with the express purpose of showing that chemicals that are tumor-producing in animals will produce mutations when applied to those particular strains (164). The conscious selection of such bacterial strains whose response supports a preconceived notion is, as was pointed out, self-fulfilling and may not be a true test of a correlation of the mutagenic and carcinogenic action of a chemical.

These and other observations, which include a partial list of not only those cancer-producing chemicals that require metabolic activation but those that act directly to induce tumors and which show no correlation between mutagenicity in the bacteria and carcinogenicity in mammalian cells, have led to the conclusion "the implication that positive results in the microbial mutagenesis system will correspond to carcinogenicity in experimental animals and humans does not appear at present to be substantiated" (164).

In comparing bacterial and mammalian cells it must also be recognized that the bacterial genome is commonly haploid while mammalian cells contain a diploid complement of chromosomes. Thus, a mutation at a single gene locus would be easily recognizable in a bacterial system while both genic alleles would have to be affected for the mutation to be dominant and, hence, easily recognizable in a mammalian system. Yet, when mammalian cells are treated in culture with carcinogenic chemicals the efficiency of conversion of such cells to tumor cells may be as high as from 3 to 20 percent (72, 165, 166) while under the best conditions may approximate 100 percent of the cell population treated (167). These figures are much higher than might reasonably be expected for randomly occurring mutations and much higher than the figures obtained when bacteria are treated with carcinogens. More meaningful insight into the mode of action of the chemical carcinogens might be obtained if the effects of a carcinogen(s) were tested for carcinogenicity and mutagenicity in the same mammalian cells under the same experimental conditions. This has now been done using freshly isolated hamster embryo cells as the experimental test object and benzo[a]pyrene or the biologically active 7,8-transdihydrodiol derivative of that compound. In that study the number of cells transformed in culture was compared with the number of mutations that occurred at a specific gene locus, the ouabain-resistance locus. The results of that study showed that 20 times more hamster cells were transformed than had mutated at the specific gene locus (168). Thus, if transformations leading to the tumorous state are due to mutations, it would be necessary to postulate the presence in mammalian systems of some extremely sensitive locus (or loci) which is specifically affected by chemical carcinogens and which under the best conditions invariably leads to the development of the tumorous state. That, if true, would be the first example (a possible exception will be considered later) of a directed mutation caused by a specific chemical in cells of higher organisms.

It should also be recalled that not only DNA but other compounds which contain electron-rich atoms in their molecules, such as the RNA's and proteins, also react with carcinogens in their ultimate active form, and the nature of the target molecule(s) in a cell that is concerned with the conversion of a normal cell to a tumor cell has by no means as yet been identified with certainty.

It is difficult for technical reasons to test the validity of the mutation hypothesis as it applies to mammalian cells. The ultimate proof could be obtained if it were possible to show that a mutant gene(s) segregates at meiosis according to the Mendelian laws of heredity. Since mammalian cells propagate themselves only vegetatively, this unequivocal test cannot be applied to them. The as yet unproved assumption that the heritable cellular changes that are commonly referred to as being mutations by cancer biologists are, in fact, mutations may, therefore, not be valid since other mechanisms may be involved.

## INDUCTION AND DETERMINATION AS ALTERNATIVE MECHANISMS TO MUTATION

The results reported above can perhaps be interpreted equally well on the basis of inductive-type mechanisms which lead to determination and ultimately to the differentiation of cells during the normal course of development. These mechanisms do not involve somatic mutations at the nuclear gene level but are concerned rather with the specific programing of the genetic information present in a cell. This type of heritable cellular change is particularly well illustrated in the case of determination and transdetermination in imaginal disc cells found in *Drosophila* larvae (169-171). These heritable cellular changes, like somatic mutations, are highly stable and the determined state may persist in a dividing population of imaginal disc cells for many years. Only when such cells are placed in a suitable environment will they differentiate into the cell type for which they have been determined. Other examples of this type of heritable cellular change were discussed in Chapter IV.

The older, extensive embryological literature dealing with so-called "nonspecific" inductive effects has shown, moreover, that substances of the most diverse type (like the cancer-producing agents), including some that have been found to be carcinogenic (estrogen) in other test systems, can act as effective inductors in early embryological development (172). Such a heritable cellular mechanism, although seldom even considered by the mutationists, provides a very real and viable alternative to the mutation hypothesis as it applies to the tumor problem. Changes of this type may be directed, often occur with high frequency, are persistent, and leave a cell potentially totipotent. Thus, although chemical carcinogens have been shown to be effective mutagens when applied not only to microorganisms but to cells of higher organisms as well, it does not necessarily follow that transformations leading to the tumorous state are the result of somatic mutations at the nuclear gene level.

All of this does not necessarily mean that the tumorous state cannot arise as a result of somatic mutation. That theory could, in principle at least, account for the origin of a tumor cell. One would, for example, have only to postulate the loss through mutation of an appropriate regulatory gene(s) (if, in fact, such genes exist in mammalian cells) to account for the unrestrained growth of a tumor cell. Nevertheless, the mutation theory has not as yet been demonstrated unequivocally to apply to any tumor system in higher animal or plant species. Since we have seen that the cancerous state may arise and be perpetuated in the presence of a complete complement of genes, any mutation that may in the future be shown to be involved in establishing the tumorous state would most probably act to persistently activate those parts of the normal cell genome that are responsible for the continued abnormal and autonomous proliferation of a tumor cell, and thus the underlying mechanism would be epigenetic in nature. This matter will be considered again later in this discussion.

# CHAPTER VI

## NATURE OF THE HERITABLE CELLULAR CHANGE, III. ADDITION OF NEW GENETIC INFORMATION

A cellular mechanism that is now well established and that has been shown to account for the origin of certain tumor cells is one that involves the addition of new genetic information resulting from infection by the tumor-inducing viruses. These oncogenic viruses represent a diverse group of disease-producing entities and, like the generality of viruses, may contain either DNA or RNA as their nucleic acid component. Although the addition of new genetic information may involve, as does somatic mutation, a change in the integrity in the chromosomal DNA of a host cell, it is basically different from somatic mutation and is commonly known as transformation. The knowledge that when new genetic information of the appropriate type is added to a cell it results in the conversion of a normal cell to a tumor cell tells us really very little about how that new information acts to bring about a heritable cellular change in the cell. In considering this matter a number of possibilities can be envisioned. The first of these is that the viral nucleic acids may serve as templates for the synthesis of new and specific proteins which are, in turn, responsible for the establishment and maintenance of the tumorous state. A second possibility that must be considered is that new and specific products derived from the activities of the viral genome may be exerting their effects indirectly by bringing about a persistent activation of those segments of the normal host cell genome that are concerned with the development of the tumorous state. Finally, the viral nucleic acids might function by means other than those involving the transcription and translation of the viral genome, and the relation of the viral nucleic acids to tumorigenesis may in certain instances be a purely physical one.

The tumor-inducing viruses, as has been indicated, represent a very heterogeneous group of disease-producing entities which may be conveniently divided for purposes of discussion into the DNA-containing viruses and the RNA-containing viruses.

## THE ONCOGENIC DNA VIRUSES

Among the most studied of the DNA-containing oncogenic viruses are the polyoma virus, the simian vacuolating virus (SV40), at least eight of the commonly found human adenoviruses, the Shope papilloma virus, as well as the herpes-type viruses. These viruses differ greatly from one another in their physical properties as well as in the types of tumors that they elicit in their hosts. For example, two papovaviruses, polyoma and SV40, are very small and contain only enough genetic information to code for about eight or so proteins, depending on their size, while herpes-type viruses and the Shope papilloma virus are much larger, contain significantly more genetic information, and hence can code for a considerably larger number of proteins. These viruses also differ greatly in the types of tumors that they induce in their hosts. Some, such as the causal agent of the Lucké adenocarcinoma of the frog, which is a herpes-type virus, are very selective as to the cell type that they transform and only the convoluted tubules of the kidney are converted into cancer cells by that virus. The Shope papilloma virus is also specific and elicits only papillomas in the skin of rabbits. While these tumors generally remain benign in their natural host, which is the wild cottontail rabbit, when that

virus is injected into the domestic rabbit it also induces the formation of papillomas but many of these benign growths develop into malignant tumors. The virus isolated from the malignant tumors has been found to be the same as that which originally produced the papillomas, suggesting that something other than the virus is responsible for the progression from the benign to the malignant state in this instance. While many of these DNA-containing viruses are highly specific not only in the type of tumor that they initiate but in the species of animal that they infect, the polyoma virus represents a dramatic exception in that it can elicit the formation of many different types of tumors in many different and unrelated species of animals. In addition to the mouse, tumors are produced by inoculation of this virus in both Chinese and Syrian hamsters, rabbits, rats, ferrets, guinea pigs, and in the multimammate mouse (*Rattis natalensis*). It has been found, further, that in one group of 117 mice inoculated soon after birth with the polyoma virus, 23 different and distinct types of tumors developed in the animals (174). Despite these findings and speculations, the most likely candidates of all of the DNA-containing viruses as causative agents of certain human cancers appear to be the herpes-type viruses. These viruses are known to cause cancers in animals; the Lucké adenocarcinoma of the frog (175) and Marek's disease of the chicken (176) are caused by viruses of the herpes type. These viruses have, moreover, commonly been found to be associated with human cancers such as, for example, cervical carcinoma, nasopharyngeal carcinomas, as well as certain lymphomas; and indirect evidence of several different types suggests that they may play an etiological role either by themselves (177) or possibly in association with certain RNA-containing viruses (178) in the initiation and development of these cancers in humans.

If we are to understand how these oncogenic viruses exert their tumorigenic effects it will be necessary for us to determine first the exact form of the association that develops between the virus and the target cell that it transforms into the tumorous state. Among the most thoroughly studied systems as far as host cell-virus interactions are concerned are those dealing with the very small, DNA-containing viruses, polyoma and SV40. The relation of these viruses to the target cell may be of two kinds which are known as productive infection and abortive infection. In the productive type of infection the virus multiplies essentially unchecked and eventually lyses and kills the infected cell. In the abortive type of infection there is little or no productive infection but there is instead a transformation leading to the development of the tumorous state. Transformations in these systems occur with low frequency in culture and only one to two percent of the cellular population treated with the virus become transformed to the tumorous state. When a cellular transformation occurs, the DNA of the virus becomes integrated into the chromosomal DNA of the host and replicates with the genome of the host cell. The viral DNA molecules are linked to the cellular DNA by alkali-stable covalent linkages (179). As indicated, no productive infection occurs in transformed cells, and hence there are no complete virus particles present in such cells. If one did not know that those cells had been transformed by a virus there would be little reason to believe that they were of viral origin. That the viral genetic information persists in such cells can be shown in a number of different ways (180, 181). One of the most convincing of these is the demonstration that when transformed cells are fused with cells of certain untransformed cell lines, the complete virus appears in the hybrid cell, indicating that all of the genetic information necessary for the production of the complete virus is retained by the transformed cells (182, 183).

The DNA of the polyoma and SV40 viruses has a molecular weight of about three million and is of a circular, double-stranded type that contains about 5000 nucleic acid bases. Since three of these bases are required to specify one amino acid, it follows that the 5000 bases can specify about 1700 amino acids. It can be calculated, moreover, from the molecular weight of the protein coat of the virus that between one-third and one-fourth of the genetic information present in the viral genome is required to specify for the viral coat protein. The remaining genetic information can specify for about 1200 amino acids, which is sufficient to code for up to eight or so new proteins. These, then, are the maximum number of viral genetic functions that can be involved in the transformation process.

Of the six, or possibly seven, viral-coded functions that have now been characterized, two appear significant as far as the transformation process is concerned. The first of these involves a viral function (gene A) that either directly or indirectly activates the synthesis of chromosomal DNA and proteins and thus removes the block that exists between the G1 and S phases of the normal cell division cycle (184-187). Evidence of several different kinds has now been presented to indicate that an intranuclear viral-coded protein, the so-called T or tumor antigen, is implicated in the initiation of chromosomal DNA synthesis in cells transformed by the SV40 virus (185, 186). The T antigen or antigens (187) could be acting directly to replace the naturally occurring cytoplasmic initiator of chromosomal DNA synthesis, or it could be acting indirectly by inducing the synthesis in transformed cells of the naturally occurring substance. Although the persistent synthesis by a cell of chromosomal DNA is clearly essential as a first step in the transformation process, that step would not in itself appear sufficient to account for the transformation as evidenced by the fact that cloned lines of cells that had been transformed by either the SV40 or the polyoma virus and that had reverted spontaneously to the "normal" state continued to produce the T antigen (145, 188). The T antigen was also found to be present in proliferating cells transformed by the SV40 virus grown under nonpermissive conditions in a temperature-sensitive system; hence the cells, although showing the normal phenotype, continued to synthesize the T antigen (186).

Another and perhaps also important virally specified function that has now been identified is one that is concerned with the presence at the surface of transformed cells of a new antigen, the so-called transplantation antigen (189, 190). This surface antigen is specific for the virus that codes for it, as evidenced by the fact that if an animal is immunized against cells transformed by the polyoma virus, it will reject cells transformed by that virus but not cells transformed by the SV40 virus. The reverse is also true. It has been found, moreover, that all tumors induced by the same virus share a common transplantation antigen and that that antigen is different for different viruses. The presence of the transplantation antigen on the surface of tumor cells may be important not only because it may reflect changes at the surface of the transformed cells which may, in turn, alter the response of those cells to regulatory influences, but because it may render those cells vulnerable to immunological attack by a host in which they are growing.

The other virally specified functions that have now been identified appear irrelevant to transformation. Thus the problem appears to be narrowly restricted to essentially two virally specified functions which may in themselves be sufficient to account for the transformation in these instances. It is also possible, since we do not know the precise role that membrane changes play in the transformation process, that additional, as yet uncharacterized, viral-specified functions concerned with later steps in the cell division cycle may be involved.

## THE ONCOGENIC RNA VIRUSES

The second group of tumor-producing viruses are those that contain RNA as their nucleic acid component. These are medium size viruses which contain a single strand of RNA that has a molecular weight of 10 to 12 million. A schematic representation of a typical RNA virus is shown in Figure 27. The most studied of these RNA-containing tumor viruses is, doubtless, the Rous sarcoma virus of chickens. The RNA of this virus has been reported to contain about 10,000 nucleotides (191, 192). Four known genetic elements have now been described as existing in the viral genome (193). These are (1) the gene(s) (*src*) responsible for sarcoma formation

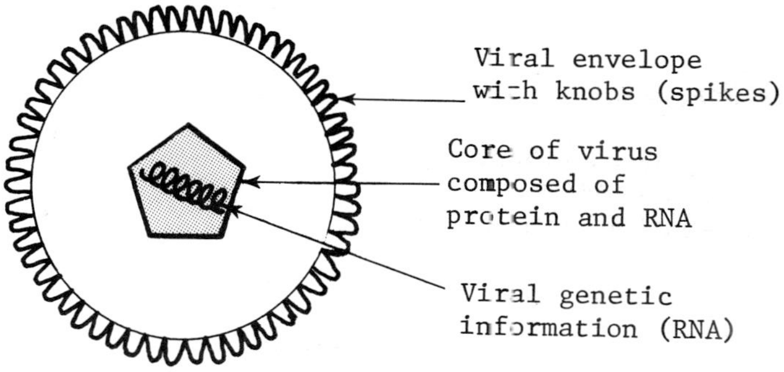


FIGURE 27. Schematic drawing of a C-type virus. Viruses of this type are commonly surrounded by an envelope. The external surface of the envelope contains many knobs or spikes. These knobs are composed of glycoproteins which serve to specifically adsorb the virus particle to the surface of the target cell. They also contain the type-specific antigen for this group of viruses. Inside the envelope is a structure known as the core shell, and found within the core is a ribonucleo protein complex which contains the genetic information of the virus.

which is composed of about 1400 nucleotides and thus constitutes about 15 percent of the total viral genetic information (194, 195); (2) the gene that codes for the group-specific antigen; (3) a gene that codes for the viral enzyme DNA polymerase; and (4) a gene that codes for viral envelope glycoprotein.

The RNA-containing viruses are very widely distributed in nature and are known to cause naturally occurring cancers in such diverse animal species as chickens, mice, and cats and are suspect in many others including man. The RNA-containing tumor viruses have been divided on the basis of their appearance into what are known as B-type particles which include the mouse and monkey mammary tumor viruses, and the C-type particles which cause, among others, the Rous sarcoma disease of chickens, leukemias and sarcomas of mice, as well as a lymphosarcoma of the cat. When C-type viruses infect appropriate cells, the viruses do not cause death of the cells, as is commonly found with other viruses, but rather cause the infected cells to proliferate actively. In contrast to the small DNA-containing viruses, the transformation from the normal to the tumorous state may occur with high frequency and commonly, as in the case, for example, of the Rous sarcoma virus, virtually all of the exposed cells in culture become transformed to the tumorous state. The infected cells, as they multiply, may or may not produce complete virus particles but in either case the viral genetic information is passed from one cell generation to the next. Other C-type and particularly B-type viruses may be far less efficient in transforming cells in culture than is the Rous sarcoma virus.

Certain of these tumor-inducing viruses behave like typical viruses in that they may be readily transmitted from a diseased to a healthy animal where they may again induce the disease. This is true of a virally-caused leukosis of chickens in which the virus has been found to be transmitted through the egg as well as by the more conventional method of contact infection from diseased to very young healthy chickens (176). Similarly, evidence is now available to show that a commonly found virally-induced lymphosarcoma of the cat may be transmitted horizontally from diseased to healthy cats and thus behaves like a typical contagious disease (196). The mammary tumor virus of the mouse is, moreover, commonly transmitted through the mother's milk and is also, therefore, a communicable disease (197).

When a virus is transmitted through the egg or the sperm from parent to offspring it is known as vertical transmission and is assumed to be the predominant route of transmission for naturally occurring leukemia-inducing viruses of the mouse.

The C-type viruses are ubiquitous and the mouse leukemia

viruses may be considered to be prototypes of this type of virus. C-type virus particles have now been reported to exist in many species of animals. They have been found to be present in cells of such diverse species as snakes, chickens, mice, cats, rats, hamsters, cattle, pigs, monkeys, apes, and man. By no means are all of these C-type viruses known to be tumor-inducing although they resemble those that do initiate tumors. For example, when mouse cells are treated with the thymidine analogues 5-bromodeoxyuridine or 5-iododeoxyuridine, a number of distinct types of previously unexpressed C-type viruses may appear (198, 199). Such viruses are known as endogenous viruses and have been found to be present in and can be induced in all mouse strains thus far tested.

The C-type viruses in mice have been studied in some detail and a new antigen, known as the group-specific antigen, was found which is specified by the virus and is common to this whole group of leukemia- and sarcoma-producing viruses. This new antigen was found to be present not only in the leukemia and sarcoma cells but was also detected in normal embryonic tissues but not in adult tissues of all mouse strains thus far studied including those believed free of either leukemia or sarcoma viruses. This finding led to the formulation of the oncogene theory of cancer which states that all adult vertebrate cells carry within their cells an unexpressed oncogenic viral genome, and that the difference between those individuals who develop cancer and those who do not is determined by whether the viral oncogene integrated in the host cell genome is expressed or repressed (200, 201). Since according to this concept the viral genome is postulated to be present but unexpressed in all cells of vertebrates, and since it is transmitted from cell to cell as a characteristic Mendelian trait, the presence of viral genes in those cells could no longer be considered abnormal since they were an intrinsic part of the normal genome of the cell. Thus, the basic cellular mechanism underlying this type of heritable cellular change would be epigenetic in nature and be similar to that found in normal development since, according to this concept, whether or not a tumor develops is determined by whether the viral oncogene present in integrated form in the host DNA is expressed or repressed.

If the oncogene theory were found to be true it would represent a generalization which could account for the development of the generality of tumors. Such cancer-producing agents as radiation and carcinogenic chemicals would simply be looked upon as being cocarcinogens that derepress and, hence, render functional a universally present oncogene. There is, moreover, now an abundance of evidence to show that lines of hamster, mice, or rat cells which do not commonly produce the complete virus can be made to do so and become transformed into tumor cells when treated with physical or chemical carcinogens.

The validity of the oncogene theory has recently been put to a rigorous test with the use of two pairs of identical human twins (202). One member of each twin pair was afflicted with acute myelocytic leukemia while the other member appeared free of the disease. If the oncogene theory is valid, then one should find identical DNA sequences in the diseased and healthy member of each twin pair since the methods used in this study detected all gene sequences whether functional or not. The results of this study showed, however, that unique leukemia-specific DNA sequences were present in the diseased member of each twin pair but absent in the healthy member, thus indicating that new leukemia-specific genetic information must have been inserted into the cellular genome following fertilization and thus argues, in this instance, against the oncogene theory. The results of this study would, nevertheless, suggest that new genetic information possibly of viral origin was inserted into the normal host cell genome and is responsible for the leukemia. It may be of interest to note here that simian sarcoma virus and baboon endogenous virus sequences have recently been detected in acute myelogenous leukemia cells of humans with the use of molecular hybridization techniques (203). The experimental findings reported in these studies would appear to be more consistent with a second theory of viral oncogenesis, the so-called provirus theory. The provirus theory postulates that the genetic information present in an oncogenic RNA virus is transcribed via an RNA-DNA hybrid into a double-stranded DNA molecule which, after being integrated into the chromosomal DNA of the host cell, may function as a template for the synthesis of viral RNA molecules and/or may function to establish and maintain the tumorous state. This theory was put on a firm experimental basis with the isolation and characterization of a new type of enzyme, an RNA-dependent DNA polymerase which was given the trivial name reverse transcriptase and which translates RNA into DNA (204, 205). This new enzyme has been found to be associated with all RNA-containing tumor viruses and with only a very few viruses not known to initiate tumors in animals. That the provirus DNA becomes integrated into, replicates with, and thus becomes an integral part of the host cell DNA is now well established experimentally (206). In addition to the oncogene and provirus hypotheses, a third theory, which is known as the protovirus hypothesis, has been proposed to account for the presence in a tumor cell of the genetic information required for the development of the tumorous state (207). According to the protovirus hypothesis, cells are postulated to contain only the potential for developing the genetic information required for the establishment and maintenance of the tumorous state. The required information is believed to arise _de novo_ as a result of multiple cycles of DNA-RNA-DNA information transfer either within cells or between cells. It has been suggested that the protovirus hypothesis may be applicable to normal developmental processes as well as to tumorigenesis. Yet, if the thesis being developed in this book, namely, that all of the genetic information necessary for the development of the tumorous state is present in the normal cell genome, is correct and that that information needs only to be persistently activated to establish the tumorous state, then it would appear quite unnecessary to postulate, as is done in the protovirus hypothesis, the _de novo_ origin of the required information through multiple cycles of DNA-RNA-DNA information transfer. The problem would resolve itself simply into learning how the new viral genetic information that is added to a cell as a result of viral infection regulates the expression of the genetic information that is normally present in a cell.

The question that arises, therefore, is: what is the specific role played by the proviral DNA in establishing and maintaining the tumorous state? Although the answer to that question is not yet in hand, it may ultimately be provided with the use of temperature-sensitive mutants of the virus. The discovery of temperature-sensitive mutants of the Rous sarcoma virus has permitted the development of experimental systems that lend themselves to meaningful studies of several different kinds (208-211). When, in those systems, chicken fibroblasts are infected with a mutant form of the Rous virus, the cells are transformed into tumor cells when incubated at a temperature of $36^{\circ}C$, which is known as the permissive temperature. These same transformed cells, when cultured at the nonpermissive temperature of $41^{\circ}C$, appear, on the other hand, perfectly normal in every respect. This temperature-sensitive process is completely and repeatedly reversible in both directions. These studies clearly demonstrate then that the genetic information present in a transformed cell and that leads to the tumorous state can be readily manipulated in these systems to give rise again to cells that show a normal phenotype. Controlled systems of this type are very useful because they permit a characterization of specific cellular changes that are either correlated with and/or etiologically involved in the transformation process. It has been reported, for example, that the inhibition of protein synthesis of cells grown at the permissive temperature, and hence showing the tumor phenotype, causes those cells to revert to the normal phenotype. The reinitiation of protein synthesis causes the reverted cells to again assume the transformed state. These results have been interpreted to mean (*a*) that protein synthesis is, as might be expected, required to maintain the transformed state, and (*b*) that the synthesis of a specific protein (the myosin-like protein referred to earlier) is not required for the cells to revert from the transformed to the normal state. Whether the normal or tumor phenotype is expressed appears to depend rather on whether the special protein is present in a cell in an ordered or disordered state (107).

That a normalization of the tumorous state may occur in the Rous sarcoma system has been convincingly demonstrated in other ways. In those studies progeny of cloned lines of hamster cells transformed by the Rous virus were plated periodically and it was found that a significant number of cells reverted from the transformed to the "normal" state (156) (see Fig. 18). Under the best conditions it was found that the revertant colonies increased in numbers from 19 percent after three weeks in culture to 98 percent after eight weeks of passage in culture. Reversions to the normal phenotype in these instances appear now to have resulted not from a loss of the proviral genome but from a persistent suppression of the proviral genetic information (212). That viral genetic information may, in fact, be lost with a resulting recovery from the tumorous state, even in those instances in which the proviral genetic information becomes an integral part of and replicates with the host cell genome, has, moreover, now been demonstrated in the case of cloned lines of cat cells transformed by the mouse sarcoma virus (213).

Although a requirement for the continued expression of all or part of the viral genome appears necessary for the establishment and maintenance of the tumorous state in the virally-induced tumors, little is as yet known about the nature of the specific products that are derived from the activity of the viral genes and that lead to the development of the tumorous state in the case of the oncogenic RNA viruses. While changes in the cellular phenotype, such as those that affect the appearance and growth habits of transformed cells as well as a reduced requirement for growth-promoting factors present in serum (214-219), increased ability to take up certain solutes from a culture medium (77-80), ability to grow as colonies in soft agar or methacel (220-222), appearance of new surface antigens and of receptor sites for the plant lectins, ability to produce and secrete into their environment proteolytic enzymes, unlimited life span *in vitro*, etc., have been found to be associated in many instances with the transformed state in culture, which one or more of these are required for the establishment and maintenance of the tumorous state is not as yet clear. This is true because cells transformed in culture do not always develop into tumorous growths when implanted into appropriate hosts, and hence a clear distinction must be made between cellular changes that accompany transformation and those involved in the establishment and maintenance of the tumorous state. This matter will be considered further later in this discussion. Phenotypic changes that characterize the transformed state in cultured cells are, nevertheless, invaluable for studying the activities of the tumor viruses.

The concept of somatic mutation and that of viral transformation both postulate persistent changes in the integrity of the genetic information present in a tumor cell. In order to be truly meaningful those postulated alterations in the host cell genome should be translated into more dynamic terms, and attempts should be made to relate those changes to specific metabolic events that underlie the tumorous state.

## THE INFLUENCE OF 5-BROMODEOXYURIDINE ON PHENOTYPIC EXPRESSION

This important problem has now been successfully approached experimentally with the use of a specific substance,

5-bromodeoxyuridine, which is a structural analogue of thymidine and which has been found to replace thymidine in the chromosomal DNA of the host cells when those cells are grown in the the presence of the analogue. 5-Bromodeoxyuridine has been used by many investigators to study different aspects of normal cellular differentiation in embryonic (223-228) as well as in certain adult cell types (229). That substance has been found to selectively suppress cellular differentiation while permitting the cell division process to proceed essentially normally. In most, but not in all, instances that have been studied, the suppression of differentiated functions by 5-bromodeoxyuridine has been found to be reversible.

It has now been reported that melanoma cells of the mouse could be made to behave in culture as do normal cells when the malignant cells were grown in the presence of appropriate concentrations of 5-bromodeoxyuridine (230). The melanoma cells, instead of piling up in random fashion characteristic of tumor cells, grew in culture as did normal cells and their growth was largely contact inhibited. The treated cells were also found to be significantly less tumorigenic when implanted into appropriate hosts than were the untreated melanoma cells. It may be of interest to note that following treatment of the melanoma cells with 5-bromodeoxyuridine a previously unrecognized endogenous C-type virus, which resembles the mouse leukemia virus, is produced in the melanoma cells (231). What role, if any, this virus plays in the etiology of the disease is not as yet known.

Several points of interest emerge from this study. The first of these is that the tumorous state, as in the case of the temperature-sensitive viral mutants, is completely and repeatedly reversible in both directions, and whether the cells behave as tumor cells or normal cells is determined by whether 5-bromodeoxyuridine is absent or present in the culture medium in which the cells are grown. A second point of interest that emerges from these studies is the finding that the decrease in tumorigenicity shown by the melanoma cells grown in the presence of 5-bromodeoxyuridine is correlated with a significant decrease in the production of a specific proteolytic enzyme, the plasminogen activator (232). We have learned earlier in this discussion that specific proteolytic enzymes play an important role in determining growth patterns expressed by cells, whether they are normal or tumor. The results of this study indicate then that the production of a specific proteolytic enzyme is associated with the malignant state, and that the suppression of that state in the melanoma system reflects an ability of 5-bromodeoxyuridine to inhibit the expression of that specialized function. Since 5-bromodeoxyuridine appears to specifically replace thymidine in the chromosomal DNA and thus bring about a change in the integrity of that DNA, this system provides a powerful tool for studying the effects of specific changes in the integrity of the DNA on the development of the tumorous state and on its reversal. Since the biosynthetic system responsible for the production of the plasminogen activator can be temporarily activated in normal cells by treating those cells with a phorbol ester, which is an active ingredient in the tumor-promoting agent croton oil, the results indicate that the plasminogen activator is coded for by host cell genes (233). The cells of the melanoma line used in these studies were heavily pigmented and synthesized melanin very efficiently. The enzyme tyrosinase catalyzes the conversion of the amino acid tyrosine to the black pigment melanin. It was found that a progressive decrease in both tyrosinase activity and melanin formation occurs during the culture of the melanoma cells in the presence of 5-bromodeoxyuridine, and cells grown continuously in a culture medium containing 5-bromodeoxyuridine showed no detectable enzyme or pigment. Thus a second specialized function coded for by host cell genes is suppressed in the melanoma cells when those cells are grown on a 5-bromodeoxyuridine-containing medium (234).

The ability of 5-bromodeoxyuridine to reversibly inhibit both the production of specific enzymes as well as tumorigenicity in melanoma cells suggests that the tumorous state in this instance, as in others, reflects the persistent activation of previously unexpressed host cell genes and, hence, is fundamentally epigenetic in nature.

# CHAPTER VII

## A SUMMARY AND SYNTHESIS

We have now reached the point in our discussion where we must try to put together our cancer puzzle and attempt a synthesis of the information that has become available to us. In considering this matter we should perhaps first ask the question whether cancer is a single disease having a common underlying cause or whether, as has often been suggested, it is a collective term used to describe more than 100 different and distinct diseases which arise in different tissues and organs, differ greatly from one another in appearance and growth habits, may follow different courses of development in their hosts, and often show different sensitivities to the different types of therapy that are applied to them. Can, in other words, the diverse manifestations of the cancerous state be accounted for on the basis of the inherent genetic potentialities that are present in but differently expressed in different types of cancers despite a common underlying cause, or does one have to postulate different and distinct underlying causes to account for the differences in the cancer phenotype that one observes? While questions of the type posed above can obviously not be answered with certainty at the present time it is, nevertheless, possible to determine whether a single underlying cellular mechanism could reasonably account for the diverse manifestations of phenotypic expression that characterizes the cancerous state.

In dealing with this matter we will attempt to find a common denominator that can account for the mode of action of the diverse physical, chemical, and biological agents that are known to convert normal cells into tumor cells and, if successful, to pinpoint where in a cell those proximate causes act to influence cellular behavior. We will choose as the central piece in our cancer puzzle, around which we must build, the now well established fact that the tumorous state can arise and be perpetuated in the presence of a complete and unaltered complement of nuclear genes. If that choice is correct, then each of the diverse bits of information that we have gathered should fall neatly into its proper place and a coherent picture of the nature of cancer should begin to emerge. The determination to use as the center piece of our puzzle the fact that the cancerous state may be established and maintained in the presence of a complete complement of nuclear genes is important because it provides a clue to the nature of the heritable cellular change that underlies the tumorous state. That information tells us that the tumor problem is fundamentally a problem of anomalous cellular differentiation and that the basic cellular mechanisms that underlie the tumorous state are similar to those that underlie differentiation that occurs during the normal course of development in all higher organisms. Both phenomena depend for their expression on a persistent activation and repression of specific but, in part, different genes present in the nucleus of a cell.

In order to now develop this thesis we must review briefly the evidence that has been presented above and upon which this concept is based. It is clear, first of all, that if an understanding of the cancer problem is ultimately to be achieved, it will be necessary for the cancer biologist to explain in mechanistic terms why tumor cells divide persistently and in an essentially unrestrained manner in their hosts, and why, in addition, cancer cells invade underlying normal tissues and metastasize to distant sites where new tumors may arise, while the growth of normal cells is precisely regulated in all higher organisms. These are dynamic problems that will ultimately find their explanations in terms of specific substances and cellular control mechanisms that are involved in the regulation of the growth of cells, tissues, and organs in an intact organism. Since the tumor problem is basically a problem of unrestrained or autonomous cell growth and division, it follows that the conversion of a normal cell to a tumor cell must involve a profound and persistent switch in the pattern of metabolism present in a cell, going from the precisely regulated metabolism that is characteristic of a normal resting cell and that is concerned with cell specialization to one involving the continued synthesis of the nucleic acids, the mitotic and enzymatic proteins, as well as the other substances that are specifically involved in continued cell proliferation which characterizes the tumorous state (235).

Several different types of experimental evidence have been presented which suggest that all of the genetic information necessary to establish and maintain the tumorous state is present in normal cells and is retained by those cells during the period that they exhibit the tumor phenotype. These include (A) the fact that normal cells of both animal and plant origin can be made to mimic perfectly for the time being the appearance and growth habits of tumor cells when treated with specific substances that do not in themselves contain genetic information. Such artificially stimulated normal cells revert to the normal phenotype when the exogenously applied stimuli are removed from the immediate environment in which such cells are growing. (B) Certain normal cell types found in both the developing embryo and in adult animals may invade normal tissues extensively and move freely through an organism and thus show certain of the fundamental attributes of cancer cells. It can reasonably be assumed that the potentialities for invasion and metastasis are inherently present but not expressed, at least not to the same degree, in most, if perhaps not all, animal cells since, as we have seen, all normal cells with very few exceptions (mature red blood cells of mammals, lens fiber cells, both of which have lost their nuclei) contain the same genetic information. Finally, (C) the demonstration in both the plant and animal fields that cells may retain during the tumorous phase all of the genetic information necessary, in the case of plant tumors, to reconstitute entirely normal fertile plants and, in the case of the teratocarcinoma of the mouse, to differentiate into most and perhaps all of the specialized cell types that make up a normal mouse. If, as the evidence now indicates, that is true, then a determination of the nature of cancer resolves itself into characterizing the regulatory mechanisms that determine which of the host cell genes are expressed or repressed and, thus, whether the normal or tumor phenotype is expressed in a cell.

What then do we know about the nature of these regulatory mechanisms? We have seen that in any proliferating population of cells, whether normal or tumor, the individual members proceed through a characteristic cycle which is composed of specific stages known as G1, S, G2, M, and D. The cell cycle is, as we have seen, regulated at each of these stages by arrest points which serve as effective breaks to prevent the unrestrained proliferation of normal cells in an organism. These arrest points in the cell cycle may be removed either by the addition of specific substances or by the removal of inhibitory substances such as the chalones. In either case, specific substances are required to remove the arrest points and, when all of the blocks have been eliminated, a cell proceeds through the cycle, divides into two daughter cells and thus completes the cycle. In a persistently dividing population of cells such as those found in tumors a mechanism(s) must exist for the persistent removal of all of the arrest points in the cell cycle. This, as we have seen, is achieved in plant tumor cells because those cells have acquired a capacity to synthesize persistently two essential growth-regulating substances which establish the pattern of synthesis concerned with cell growth and division. Since these two growth-regulating substances are produced persistently by plant tumor cells, their continued presence in those cells maintains that pattern of synthesis in the cells. While those two substances acting together remove persistently all of the arrest points that regulate the normal cell cycle, other substances needed for the synthesis of the nucleic acids, the mitotic and enzymatic proteins, etc., which have now been largely identified in plant tumor systems, must also be synthesized persistently by the tumor cells if the pattern of synthesis concerned with continued cell growth and division is to be expressed.

Since precisely the same arrest points exist in the cell cycle of animal cells as have been described for plant cells, it would seem reasonable to assume that similar underlying cellular mechanisms, although not necessarily the same substances, are involved in removing the blocks that exist in the animal cell cycle. Experimental evidence presented earlier in this discussion suggests that this may, in fact, be true. It has long been known that a cytoplasmic initiator of chromosomal DNA synthesis exists in animal cells and this substance has been found in organisms that are as taxonomically different as the protozoa and the vertebrates. A substance that initiates chromosomal DNA synthesis and which appears to be a protein having a molecular weight of about 50,000 has now been isolated from mammalian cells. This substance, like the initiator of chromosomal DNA synthesis in plants, removes the G1 phase block in the normal cell cycle. Other studies have reported that a second substance, also apparently a protein, acts synergistically with the first to promote cell division in certain animal cell types. This second protein, like the cell-division-promoting factor in plants, is ineffective in triggering either DNA synthesis or cell division in the absence of the factor that initiates chromosomal DNA synthesis. If additional work in this area confirms the suggestions that two substances acting together remove all of the blocks in the animal cell cycle, then the continued production by a cell of those two growth-regulating substances could account, in large part at least, for the continued abnormal and autonomous proliferation of an animal tumor cell. If that concept is correct, then one should find these two substances to be absent in normal resting cells, to be present during specific stages of the cell cycle in normal cells that have been stimulated to divide, and absent in those cells when the stimulus is withdrawn and cell division stops while they should be synthesized persistently by dividing animal tumor cells. According to this view the substances that remove the blocks in the normal cell cycle are the same as those that perform a similar function in tumor cells, and whether the biosynthetic systems that produce those substances are under precise regulation or whether they are persistently activated determines in large part whether or not a cell will grow in an autonomous manner in its host. It is, of course, possible in certain select instances that the naturally occurring cytoplasmic initiator of chromosomal DNA synthesis may be replaced by a substance that is, for example, coded for by viral genetic information. It has been reported that the T antigen, which is specified by genetic information present in the SV40 and polyoma viruses, initiates chromosomal DNA synthesis in cells transformed by those viruses. Thus either the T antigen may replace the naturally occurring initiator of chromosomal DNA synthesis or the presence of that virally-coded protein in a cell induces the cell to synthesize the naturally occurring initiator of chromosomal DNA synthesis.

If the basic concept outlined above is correct, then the question might reasonably be asked why certain cells transformed in culture by physical, chemical, or biological agents may appear by all generally accepted criteria to be tumorous, and yet, when those cells are implanted into appropriate hosts they do not develop into tumorous growths. There appear to be a number of possible reasons for this. One of the most obvious is that because of the presence of new surface properties on the transformed cells, those cells are recognized by the host as foreign bodies and are thus rejected. It is also possible that certain of the transformed cells in culture are incompletely transformed in the sense that those cells have not acquired an ability to synthesize all of the essential factors required for their continued growth in a host. The culture medium in which such transformants are grown is often very complex and contains readily available substances of many different kinds that are required for the growth of cells. Thus, conditionally transformed cells may obtain one or more of the essential growth substances from the culture medium that they require for growth but cannot themselves make. When such cells are implanted into a host, that substance(s) is not readily available and hence such cells do not develop into a tumorous growth. There are many examples which illustrate that this may, in fact, be true. We have seen that during the transition from a normal plant cell to a fully autonomous, rapidly growing tumor cell a series of quite distinct but well defined biosynthetic systems, which represent the entire area of cellular metabolism concerned with cell growth and division, become progressively and persistently activated and the degree of activation of those systems within a cell determines the rate of growth of the tumor cell. We have seen, moreover, that the individual biosynthetic systems can be activated independently of one another or they can all be activated more or less simultaneously. If, for example, all of the necessary biosynthetic systems except the auxin system are persistently activated in a plant cell that cell will not grow unless an exogenous source of the plant growth hormone auxin is supplied to such partially transformed cells. Those cells thus behave as hormone-dependent tumor cells although they may and frequently do acquire a capacity to synthesize their own hormone during later periods of their growth and then become true tumor cells. What appears to be an entirely comparable situation, differing only in particulars, is found in the case of the conditional or hormone-dependent tumors of animals and humans. There are, in addition, conditionally transformed animal cells which when implanted into appropriate hosts develop into tumors only when those cells are attached to glass beads (236). Tumorigenicity in these instances is anchorage-dependent, a trait which is lost when those same cells become fully transformed to the tumorous state. A similar situation may exist during the transition from the benign to the malignant state when newly expressed traits such as an ability to invade and/or metastasize may be acquired by the originally benign tumor cells. That a persistent derepression of biosynthetic systems may be very extensive and go well beyond those required for establishing the tumorous state is evidenced by the numerous examples in which tumor cells have acquired an ability to synthesize specific substances that the cell types from which those tumors arose do not commonly produce. It has been found, for example, that liver tumor cells contain an antigen which is identical to one present in embryonic or fetal liver tissue but is not found in normal adult liver cells (237). Similar results have been obtained with human gastrointestinal tumors (238, 239). The results of these studies indicate then that genetic information that was expressed in the embryo or fetus was subsequently repressed following the differentiation of the liver or gastrointestinal cells and was again expressed in cancer cells derived from those cell types. Numerous other examples of this type have been reviewed in the literature (240, 241) including the production of an ACTH-like substance by a primary carcinoma of the lung (242) and gonadotrophin by a bronchogenic carcinoma (243). It is clear, therefore, that, as a result of the conversion of normal cells to tumor cells, the tumor cells may acquire biosynthetic capacities that are not expressed in their mature normal counterparts, indicating that an extensive and persistent derepression of the normal cellular genome may occur during the tumor transformation process.

All of these studies suggest then that the tumorous state and various manifestations of that state result from a persistent activation of normally repressed biosynthetic systems, the products of which are required not only for the establishment and maintenance of the tumorous state but to give different kinds of tumor cells their characteristic properties. Since cells of all higher organisms contain thousands of different genes many of which code for different traits, it should not be surprising to find that cells of different tumors, even those derived from the same tissues, may exhibit quite different characteristics depending upon which of the genes are active and which are repressed and, hence, nonfunctional. Thus cancer, from a biological point of view, could be considered to be a single disease (rather than a multiplicity of diseases) in which the diverse manifestations of the tumorous state commonly observed would simply reflect different expressions of a common underlying cellular mechanism.

What then are the factors that activate the synthesis in cells of the substances that remove the arrest points in the normal cell cycle, and what are the cellular mechanisms that regulate the production of those factors in a cell? While the cell division process is now understood, in broad outline at least, in higher plant species in the sense that that process can be completely controlled under precisely defined experimental conditions with the use of specific naturally occurring substances, that process is not as well understood in cells of higher animals although some clues are now beginning to emerge. We have seen that proteolytic enzymes (e.g., the overgrowth-stimulating factor) are produced by certain tumor cells and that those enzymes may exert profound effects on certain normal cell types causing those cells to assume for the time being the appearance and growth habits of tumor cells. The proteolytic enzymes probably exert their growth-promoting effects by altering temporarily the properties of the plasma membranes that form the outer surface of the cells. It has been indicated that two proteins, one a protease known as the plasminogen activator and which is secreted by transformed cells while the other, plasminogen, is a component of serum, interact to give rise to the enzyme fibrinolysin which digests fibrin. Although normal cells treated with proteolytic enzymes may show certain characteristic properties of tumor cells, those enzymes appear, for reasons presented earlier, to be more specifically concerned with an ability of cancer cells to migrate than with a capacity of those cells to grow in an autonomous manner. An as yet incompletely characterized "migration factor" has, moreover, now been isolated from certain cancer cells which could play an important role in conferring on those cells a capacity for invasion and metastasis. A protein-containing substance that is produced by certain normal cells has also been isolated which, when applied to certain highly malignant cells in culture, restores contact inhibition of growth in the malignant cell types and causes those cells to behave in culture in this respect as do normal cells. Thus, both the capacities for migration as well as for contact inhibition of growth appear, in these instances at least, to be controlled by specific substances. Insight into the manner by which these biologically active substances are regulated in a cell is clearly important to an understanding of the tumor problem.

The role of specific inorganic ions in the regulation of cell growth and division in both the plant and animal fields has been indicated earlier in this discussion. This is particularly well illustrated by the demonstration of the role that the $Ca^{++}$ ion plays in the regulation of the normal cell division cycle and the relative independence of all cancer cells thus far studied for that ion during cell proliferation. The $Mg^{++}$ ion has also been found to be an essential cofactor required for the activity of the initiator of chromosomal DNA synthesis and thus, like the $Ca^{++}$ ion, assists in removing the block that exists in the G1 stage of the cell cycle.

While studies of the type described above provide us with clues to why tumor cells proliferate in an essentially unrestrained or autonomous manner in their hosts, they do not tell us whether the heritable cellular changes that underlie the tumorous state are of a permanent and irreversible type or whether those changes are potentially reversible in the generality of tumors. We have seen that a persistent suppression of or a recovery from the tumorous state leading to a normalization of the tumor phenotype may occur in cells present in a wide spectrum of tumors that range in origin, on the one hand, from those found in higher plant species to select cancers that develop in man, on the other. Since tumors that show potentialities for reversibility may be initiated by diverse physical, chemical, and biological agents, the results obtained in these studies would appear to have broad biological implications. Yet, it is argued by some that examples of the type used to illustrate the potential reversibility of the tumorous state represent special cases and do not necessarily apply to the generality of tumors. The concept of the irreversibility of the tumorous state had over the years become so thoroughly ingrained in the thinking of cancer pathologists that it had become accepted dogma which very few ever questioned. The author was repeatedly assured some few years ago by a very eminent experimental oncologist that, while animal tumor cells may and frequently do progress from "bad to worse" during the course of their development, a reversion from the tumorous to the nontumorous state does not appear to occur in animal tumor systems. It was his considered opinion that plant tumor systems were perhaps unique in that respect. This assertion was made despite the fact that the oncologist had studied in some detail, and over a considerable period of time, a transplantable keratoma of the mouse the bulk of the cells of which, although apparently derived from actively dividing tumor cells, had become terminally differentiated and had lost their tumorous properties. It should perhaps be emphasized here that simply because the generality of tumor cells behave as though they were irreversibly altered cells is clearly not in itself sufficient reason for believing that they are, in fact, irreversibly altered cells.

While it is, of course, not as yet possible for technical reasons to determine whether the generality of tumor cells are irreversibly altered or whether they are potentially reversible, it is, nevertheless, now possible in certain select instances to test this question experimentally. The Lucké adenocarcinomas of the leopard frog appear by all generally accepted criteria to be composed of irreversibly altered cells which behave in all essential respects as do cancer cells generally. Yet, it will be recalled that when a cancer nucleus of Lucké adenocarcinoma cells is isolated and injected into an activated but enucleated normal frog egg, the cancer nucleus directs perfectly normal development to proceed to the tadpole stage. The tadpoles that developed from the cancer-derived nuclei showed no evidence of malignancy and they contained all of the specialized cell types, tissues, and organs found in normal tadpoles in the same stage of development. It seems apparent, therefore, that those cytoplasmic factors and regulatory mechanisms that are present in normal frog eggs and that are known from extensive embryological studies to program a normal nucleus in a very precise and highly predictable manner during the normal course of development can also reprogram the genetic information present in a cancer nucleus in such a way as to permit normal development to proceed to the tadpole stage. A characterization of the cytoplasmic factors and regulatory mechanisms that direct development is clearly a most important consideration for an understanding of the cancer problem. It seems not unlikely that the generality of cancer cell nuclei might behave similarly if they could be subjected to the same type of experimental approach.

It was because of the truly unique characteristics of not only the Lucké system but of the other test systems in which a reversal of the tumorous state was demonstrable experimentally that the possibility of reprograming of the genetic information present in a tumor cell nucleus could be approached in such a direct manner with so definitive an answer. It does not seem very profitable to argue, at least not until sound experimental evidence is provided, that the experimental test systems that have been used to demonstrate the reversibility of the tumorous state somehow represent curious exceptions and that information obtained with the use of such systems may not be applicable to the generality of tumors. It is often and sometimes only through the use of novel experimental approaches of the type described above that meaningful insight can be gained into complex biological phenomena such as cancer.

A demonstration of the reprograming of the genetic information present in the nucleus of a cancer cell is not confined to experimental test systems that are manipulated under laboratory conditions but it occurs naturally and spontaneously although apparently rarely in patients afflicted with certain advanced malignancies. Mention was made earlier of the neuroblastomas of humans in which a significant number of very well documented instances have been recorded in the literature in which complete regressions of advanced metastasizing neuroblastomas occurred. The basis of these regressions was not death of the neuroblastoma cells or their rejection by the host but was due rather to their maturation and differentiation into ganglion cells that had lost their malignant properties. Patients in whom such regressions occurred lived for many years without recurrence of the malignant tumor. It is clearly important to determine the basis of such regressions for, if the reasons underlying them were understood, it could well lead to a useful approach for the control of this highly malignant disease. While those mechanisms are not as yet understood, some progress has been made in inducing the maturation in culture of neuroblastoma cells with the use of specific substances such as the nerve growth factor and dimethylsulfoxide. Dimethylsulfoxide has also been found to induce in culture the maturation and differentiation of erythroleukemic cells of the mouse. This substance is known to greatly facilitate the movement of substances of many kinds into cells from their immediate environment. Mention was also made earlier in this discussion of a naturally occurring, inducing substance which, when applied to acute myelocytic leukemic cells of humans in culture, causes those cells to mature into granulocytes and macrophages that have lost their malignant properties. This substance appears to be required for the maturation of normal granulocytes and macrophages from their immature progenitor cells in a normal intact organism. Another class of nontoxic tissue-specific substances that can profoundly influence phenotypic expression are the chalones. These substances inhibit cell division and by doing so encourage differentiation of many different normal cell types (244). Finally, we have seen that the stable, biologically active 8-bromo derivative of cyclic AMP(3'5') causes plant cells to differentiate into tracheary elements, and when this happens in plant tumor cells those cells become terminally differentiated with a loss of their neoplastic properties.

The results of all of these studies indicate then that cells present in many different tumors found in a wide spectrum of organisms may retain, during the time that they exhibit the tumor phenotype, a capacity to mature and differentiate with a loss of their tumorous properties. All of the genetic information necessary to code for the specific types of differentiation is clearly retained in these instances by the tumor cells. The specific substances that have been shown to encourage the maturation and differentiation of the tumor cells appear to act by removing a block for differentiation that exists in those cells, thus permitting the cells to again fully express their characteristic specialized functions.

Certain of the tumor systems described above that have been shown to be reversible involve a change in the integrity of the genetic information present in a cell or are presumed to result from such a change. The Lucké adenocarcinoma of the frog and Friend's erythroleukemia of the mouse are caused by oncogenic viruses and the addition and integration of new viral genetic information into the host cell genome is involved in these instances. The epidermoid (squamous) carcinoma is, on the other hand, readily induced in experimental animals with ionizing radiation and because of this is presumed by some to result from damage to the chromosomal DNA. Yet, in these instances a reversal of the tumorous state has been demonstrated to occur. Let us turn next to other experimental test systems in which a change in the integrity of the genetic information present in the nucleus of a cell and that leads to the development of the tumorous state has either been demonstrated to occur or is assumed by some to occur. We have seen that viral genetic information may become integrated directly by means of covalent linkages into a host cell genome in the case of the DNA-containing oncogenic viruses, or in the form of a DNA provirus in the case of the oncogenic RNA viruses. In either case the viral genetic information is transmitted from cell to cell as an integral part of the host cell DNA. The integrated viral genetic information may, as we have seen, be present and expressed, leading to the development of the tumor phenotype, or it may be present but suppressed, giving rise to cells that show the normal phenotype. The integrated viral genes may thus be regulated in a cell in much the same manner as are other parts of the host cell genome and appear to be subject to many of the same regulatory mechanisms that influence the activity of the normal chromosomal genes. The regulation of viral genetic information appears to be particularly well illustrated in the case of the temperature-sensitive viral mutants in which a few degrees difference in the temperature at which the transformed cells are incubated determines whether the normal or tumor phenotype is expressed. Thus, the cellular mechanism that underlies viral transformations appears to be epigenetic in nature since whether the normal phenotype or the tumor phenotype is expressed is determined by whether select genes in the chromosomal DNA are active or silent.

The effect of a change in the integrity of the genetic information present in a cell on the determination of phenotypic expression is illustrated further in the case of a highly malignant melanoma cell of the mouse. When cells of this melanoma are treated in culture with the thymidine analogue 5-bromodeoxyuridine they grow as do normal cells. Since 5-bromodeoxyuridine in this instance very probably replaces thymidine in the host DNA, as it has been shown to do in other systems, we are dealing here with a highly specific but readily reversible change in the integrity (involving base substitutions) of the genetic information present in a cell. Thus, whether the melanoma cells grow as normal cells or as cancer cells is determined by whether 5-bromodeoxyuridine is present or absent in the culture medium in which the melanoma cells are grown. It has been found, moreover, that whether the normal phenotype or the tumor phenotype is expressed is correlated with an ability of the cells to produce a specific proteolytic enzyme, the plasminogen activator. We have seen that the growth pattern and behavior of certain normal cell types in culture is greatly influenced by proteolytic enzymes. Thus, when the melanoma cells produce the plasminogen activator they exhibit the malignant phenotype, while when those same cells are grown in the presence of 5-bromodeoxyuridine they fail to produce the enzyme and behave in culture as do normal cells. It was pointed out, moreover, that the biosynthetic system that produces that enzyme in normal cells can be temporarily activated by treating those cells with certain phorbol esters, which are the active ingredients of the tumor-promoting substance croton oil. This finding indicates that the plasminogen activator is coded for by host cell genes. A second enzyme, tyrosinase, which also is coded for by host cell genes, is functional in melanoma cells and is involved in the conversion of tyrosine into melanin which, in turn, gives those cells their characteristic black color. The synthesis of this enzyme, like the plasminogen activator, is suppressed when the melanoma cells are grown in the presence of 5-bromodeoxyuridine and assume the normal phenotype. These findings suggest that even in those instances in which changes occur in the integrity of the genetic information that is normally present in a cell, the fate of the cell is determined by whether specific host cell genes are active or suppressed. Thus, if the tumorous state should ultimately be shown in some or even in many instances to result from somatic mutation, the mutant gene(s) would probably act via epigenetic mechanisms to persistently alter the expression of those parts of the normal cell genome that are responsible for the establishment and maintenance of the tumorous state.

Finally, we have seen that in those few instances in which a meaningful analysis of the relationship between abnormal chromosome numbers in a cell and the tumorous state has been made, the results suggest that here, too, the underlying mechanism is fundamentally epigenetic in nature.

It thus appears that the heritable cellular change that underlies the tumorous state generally, like that found in normal development, is epigenetic in nature and depends for its expression on a persistent activation and/or repression of select genes present in the chromosomes of a cell. The diverse physical, chemical, and biological agents known to initiate tumors are all apparently capable of achieving this same end result, as are the persistent switches in the patterns of metabolism that occur spontaneously in the absence of any recognizable tumor-inducing agent. This, then, appears to be the point in a cell in which all of the proximate causes meet and it is here that attention should be focused.

The results of all of the studies reviewed above suggest then that cells present in a wide spectrum of organisms retain during the tumorous phase all of the genetic information required to reconstitute the normal phenotype. So broad, in fact, is this spectrum of examples now that it is tempting to assume that this is a characteristic of the generality of tumors. If that is true, then the cancer problem resolves itself into learning how the genetic information is regulated in a cell to give rise, on the one hand, to the tumor phenotype and, on the other, the normal phenotype. The possible cellular control systems that could be involved in determining phenotypic expression are varied and could function in a cell at either the transcriptional level, the translational level, or both. It is, nevertheless, true, and this is the important point, that nuclear gene function is not irreversibly fixed in a cell and can certainly no longer now be considered to be beyond hope of correction. We have seen that an interphase nucleus is highly responsive to the environmental conditions in which it operates and factors such as wounding and other forms of stress, certain hormonal stimuli, changes in nutrition, specific inorganic ions, inductive stimuli, as well as the cytoplasmic factors that have been found to play a central role in the regulation of both the cell division process and in cell differentiation can profoundly influence nuclear gene activity. Thus, superimposed on the gene action system are mechanisms whereby the transcription and/or the translation of the genetic information present in a cell are made conditional on specific stimuli. It has, however, now become abundantly clear that the regulation of gene expression is exceedingly complex and that many different types of control mechanisms may be involved. All of these regulatory mechanisms must, nevertheless, ultimately converge on or profoundly influence, either directly or indirectly, the expression of nuclear gene activity. Mention was briefly made earlier in this discussion of control mechanisms that have now been well characterized and that play an important role in the regulation of bacterial metabolism. These have been reviewed in detail elsewhere and will not be dealt with further here (245-247).

In considering the matter of gene regulation at another level it should be recalled that the chromosomal DNA is present either in an active or diffuse state or in an inactive or condensed state. This suggests that the physical state of the DNA is somehow determined by other chromosomal constituents.

In addition to DNA, two general classes of proteins, (A) the basic proteins or histones and (B) the nonhistone or acidic proteins, as well as RNA's are found associated with the chromosomes. The histones present in the chromosomes of animals and plants have been classified into five main groups. These groups differ from one another in a number of respects but most strikingly perhaps in their contents of two basic amino acids, arginine and lysine. The lysine-rich histones have most commonly been found associated with the inert chromosomes or condensed regions of chromosomes, while the arginine-rich histones have been found to be associated with the diffuse or RNA-synthesizing regions of the chromosomes. The physical state of the histones within the chromosomes may be modified further through methylation, acetylation, and phosphorylation. These proteins may thus show structural modifications which can in certain instances be correlated with functional activity (248, 249). In this regard acetylation appears particularly interesting because it has been found to occur selectively in certain of the histones just before the time of active RNA synthesis at given gene loci.

This type of acetylation is not in itself sufficient, however, to start transcription but appears rather to be somehow concerned with changing the physical state of the chromatin so as to make the DNA available for transcription. While the histones must obviously be considered in any attempt to explain the functioning of chromatin, they appear to lack both the specificity and the diversity required to account for the selective activation and repression of the thousands of different genes that give different cell types their characteristic properties. More promising candidates as providers of the necessary specificity for switching genes present in a cell on and off are the nonhistone or acidic proteins present in the chromosomes (250). These proteins, in contrast to the histones, represent a highly diverse group of substances and, again in contrast with the histones, their concentration has been found to increase at sites of active gene transcription. Although the precise mechanism by which these acidic proteins interact with the genome to initiate, augment, or otherwise modify the transcription of specific mRNA molecules has not as yet been resolved, experimental evidence has been presented to suggest that gene regulation may involve a nonhistone protein-DNA interaction by a selective phosphorylation and dephosphorylation of the nonhistone protein (251). Nevertheless, what appears to be required is a control mechanism that permits gene recognition by complementary base-pairing between the DNA nucleotides of the cellular genome and a complementary nucleotide sequence (252, 253). Such a control mechanism would offer an attractive alternative to the view that proteins alone recognize and influence the function of genetic loci in a chromosome. Such a hypothetical control mechanism might involve the delivery and binding of regulatory proteins at sites in the cellular genome dictated by the recognition sequences of attached RNA nucleotides. The low molecular RNAs that have been reported to be associated with chromosomal proteins might provide such a regulatory mechanism.

Before concluding this section, mention should perhaps be made of possible mechanisms that could explain how changes in gene expression can be perpetuated in a stable fashion in a persistently dividing population of cells and in the presence of a constant cellular genome. For a recent discussion of possible mechanisms that may be involved, the reader is referred to reference number 61, pages 101-105 and the references that are cited therein.

Essentially two general classes of mechanisms that could account for the stability of phenotypic expression have been suggested. These are, firstly, the so-called template theories, of which cytotaxis or cortical inheritance in *Paramecium* is a much studied example. This type of mechanism illustrates how patterns of development are determined, in certain instances at least, by pre-existing structures. Thus, although the properties of pattern-forming systems are genetically determined, the expression of the actual pattern that forms is determined by the arrangement of pre-existing structure. There is as yet no evidence for the etiological involvement of pattern inheritance in the neoplastic transformation.

A second general class of mechanisms that could account for the stability of the tumorous state in a dividing population of cells and in the presence of a constant cellular genome are the so-called steady-state theories. Certain of these theories assume that alternative steady states exist in cellular metabolism and that those states are regulated by either negative or positive feedback mechanisms. A number of rather ingenious models which could, in principle at least, account for the stability of phenotypic expression in a dividing population of cells have been devised. That regulatory systems of this type may, in fact, be importantly involved in the control of gene expression in certain tumors is evidenced by the fact that mechanisms based on feedback control have now been shown to regulate the production of certain essential growth-promoting substances in plant tumor cells (119).

Whatever the ultimate mechanism(s) for gene regulation for the generality of tumor cells will turn out to be, it is nevertheless clear that if we are going to be able to manipulate nuclear gene function at will those mechanisms will have to be understood. An understanding of those regulatory mechanisms will not only yield the desired insight but could well ultimately provide alternative and perhaps more rational methods of control than are now being used for the treatment of certain cancers. We now appear to be at the very beginning of an understanding of the factors and regulatory mechanisms required to accomplish that end. This is an area of cancer biology that has until recently been largely neglected. It is, nevertheless, one that will have to be explored in depth if we are really to understand the cancer problem.

# CHAPTER VIII

# THE PREVENTION, DETECTION, AND TREATMENT OF CANCER

We have attempted in the foregoing discussion to characterize cancer as a biological problem and thus provide insight into our present understanding of the nature of that disease. Since cancer is an urgent public health problem, it would seem appropriate to examine next the practical aspects of that problem to learn what is now being done and what might possibly be done in the future to deal with that disease.

## GEOGRAPHICAL DISTRIBUTION

That striking differences in the incidence of certain cancers may occur from one country to another as well as in different parts of the same country has long been known. For example, in Japan (as well as in Scandinavia) the incidence of stomach cancer is high. Breast cancer among Japanese, Chinese, and American Indian women is, on the other hand, low. The opposite is true among white Americans. Cancer of the colon in Japan is rare but the incidence increases significantly among Japanese who move to Hawaii or to the mainland of the United States where they may consume a more typical American diet. The incidence of liver cancer, on the other hand, is very high in certain parts of equatorial Africa while among Americans including those of African descent it is, by comparison, relatively low. The high incidence of cancer of the liver in Africa has been correlated with the eating of foodstuffs, particularly peanuts, which have become contaminated with aflatoxins. The aflatoxins are highly carcinogenic products of the fungus Aspergillus flavus and they may be found in foodstuffs that are stored under warm, moist conditions.

Perhaps the most comprehensive study that has yet been made on the relationship that exists between cancer incidence and geography in a single country is found in the recently published report by scientists of the National Center for Health Statistics of the U.S. Department of Health, Education, and Welfare. This twenty-year study, published in 1975 under the title "Atlas of Cancer Mortality for U.S. Counties 1950-1969," provides data on type of cancers, age, race, sex, and place of residence. It was assumed, moreover, in this study that similar distribution patterns for specific cancers in both men and women would indicate that some common environmental factor(s) was involved, while marked differences in those patterns in the sexes would tend to implicate occupational factors. Some of the findings resulting from such mappings are listed below.

A high incidence of lung cancer was reported not only in urban industrial areas of the country but also along the Gulf Coast from Texas and Louisiana to the Florida panhandle, as well as along the Atlantic Coast from northern Florida to Charleston, South Carolina, suggesting that environmental factors in addition to cigarette smoking may contribute to lung cancer in these essentially rural and seaport areas. Melanomas were found, moreover, to be far more prevalent in the southern United States where prolonged exposure to strong sunlight is most marked.

The incidence of stomach cancers, on the other hand, was high in both sexes in the north central States and corresponds to the area of the country where persons of Scandinavian descent are concentrated. In the northeastern States a higher than average incidence of oral cancers as well as of cancers of the bladder were found but only in males, suggesting the influence of occupational factors in these instances. Cancers of the colon and rectum in both sexes were found to be significantly more prevalent in the northern States than in the southern or in the central States. The results of all of these studies suggest then that environmental influences such as diet, air and water environments, differences in life styles, occupations, as well as hereditary factors may play a most important role in determining cancer incidence.

## PREVENTION OF CANCER

Since an estimated 70 percent or more of all human cancers are caused by environmental hazards, it is clearly imperative, as a first step, to identify those cancer-producing agents and eliminate them from the environment insofar as that is possible in modern industrial societies. Prevention is unquestionably the most effective way of dealing with cancer at the present time.

There are, in addition to the environmental influences to which the general population is exposed, those individuals who, because of their occupations, run a far greater than normal risk of developing cancers. Mention has already been made of the chimney sweeps who developed scrotal cancers, workers in the aniline dye industry who developed bladder cancers, those who mined or worked with asbestos or those who inhaled dust from chromate ores developed lung cancer, while workers in nickel-refining plants developed cancers of the nasal sinuses. There are many other well documented instances of occupational cancers. One of these involves the women who painted luminous dials on watches by dipping their brushes into a dilute radium-containing solution and then pointing those brushes in their mouths. Many developed osteosarcomas (cancer of the bone) as a result of the prolonged use of this practice. A recent and much publicized example is found in the case of workers in the plastic industry who were exposed to vinyl chloride, a gaseous chemical widely used in that industry. Two dozen or so workers in several plastics manufacturing plants have developed a rare tumor of the liver known as an angiosarcoma. Since the number of workers that developed these tumors represents only a very small proportion of the total number of workers in those plants, it is unlikely that a causal relationship would have been established in this instance if the tumors that developed had been of a more commonly found type. These are but a few of the many examples of this type which, once recognized, either have been or could be avoided by discontinuing the practice or by using proper protective measures.

It is estimated that more than 30,000 chemicals have come into commercial production and have thus become widely distributed in the past and this list grows by more than 1,000 each year. Many of these have, needless to say, not been tested adequately for their cancer-producing capacities. It is imperative therefore that rapid, reliable, and inexpensive methods be developed for screening compounds for their potential carcinogenic properties. This is particularly true because certain cancers such as those that develop, for example, in the lungs or in the colon may show latent periods of from 20 to as long as 30 years. Thus, cancers that are now being diagnosed clinically may, in fact, have originated some two or three decades ago. This emphasizes the urgent need for recognizing and eliminating cancer-producing substances from the environment now so that an epidemic of cancers may not occur in the future.

Of the approximately 1,000 compounds that have now been shown to induce the formation of tumors in experimental animals some 30 are definitely known to cause cancers in humans. This, then, raises the question as to what criteria should be applied to decide whether any given substance is or is not carcinogenic for humans. This question is not always easy to resolve. While it is perhaps true that all substances that are known to cause cancers in humans have also been found to produce cancers when applied to one or another species of animals, by no means all agents that have been found to cause cancers in animals have been shown to be carcinogenic in humans. Many variables are involved in studies of this type including, among others, not only the species of experimental animals being used to conduct the studies but whether inbred lines of a given species are inherently high or low cancer-producing strains.

There is now a growing controversy developing over the guidelines that should be used in making these determinations. There are, on the one hand, the environmentalists who believe that any substance that causes tumors in animals or, for that matter, in living tissue of any kind should be characterized as being carcinogenic and, hence, a hazard to humans. They often advocate zero tolerance and argue for the complete elimination of those substances from the environment. The other group, the pragmatists, insist that those criteria are much too restrictive and believe that a compromise is necessary. They argue that the potential health hazard of a substance must be weighed against its overall benefit to mankind.

The development of rapid, reliable, and inexpensive methods for detecting cancer-inducing properties of compounds would appear to be a most important priority in the battle against cancer. The methods that have in the past been used and are now being developed for screening potential cancer-producing substances can be divided roughly into two broad categories which include, on the one hand, the use of whole animals and, on the other, the so-called sub-mammalian assay systems. The use of whole animals as test organisms is perhaps the most reliable method now available because if carried out properly it has a high predictive value. However, it is a very expensive and time-consuming method that, from a practical point of view, permits the screening of only a relatively few of the thousands of substances that may have potential cancer-producing properties. It is estimated that in order to get statistically significant results, particularly when weakly carcinogenic substances are involved, a minimum of 455 animals should be used for testing each substance and the test animals must be maintained throughout their life span which, in the case of a mouse, may be two years or more. It is clear that if large numbers of compounds are to be tested, much faster and cheaper methods for screening are required. Several such systems which show promise are now under active investigation. One of these is a method whereby the cancer-inducing properties of a substance are tested directly in culture on isolated mammalian cells. Of these, the experimental test systems using fibroblasts are most advanced but because of the poor ability of those cell types to metabolize carcinogens into their ultimate active forms it is necessary to supplement the fibroblast cultures with enzymes required to accomplish this conversion. While the only valid method for determing whether the conversion from the normal to the tumorous state has been accomplished in culture is to implant treated cells into appropriate hosts and learn whether tumors will develop from the implanted cells, the criteria for transformation used in many of these studies have depended on secondary characteristics such as, for example, the ability of cells to form colonies in soft agar or to grow in random fashion on the surface of an agar medium, etc. As indicated earlier, these criteria may not in themselves be adequate for establishing whether a conversion to the tumorous state has occurred. These methods, if now developed and refined further, nevertheless, appear to offer promise as potential rapid screening systems for chemical carcinogens.

Other methods that are now receiving a great deal of attention and that are very inexpensive to carry out, yield information in short periods of time, and for which a high predictability is claimed are those that equate damage to the chromosomal DNA with carcinogenicity. These methods use bacterial species such as, for example, mutant strains of *Salmonella typhimurium* as the experimental test object and, in one of the most commonly used of these assays, measure DNA damage by determining mutation rates in the test organisms. Although 90 percent predictability is claimed in these studies, false positives and false negatives are encountered and some of these have been referred to in Chapter V. Microbial systems which depend on other characteristics such as, for example, rate of or ability to repair DNA damage and which utilize bacterial species such as *Escherichia coli* and *Bacillus subtilis* are also being studied. These microbial systems are now being investigated to learn their usefulness as first-tier screening methods. It is, nevertheless, generally agreed that in their present state of development no one method should be relied upon and that several should be used for each compound tested to eliminate as far as possible the false positives and false negatives that may be encountered.

In addition to the environmental hazards that the general population, particularly those living in urban industrial societies, are regularly exposed to and the cancers that are largely confined to those working in certain occupations, there are those hazards that are self-inflicted and result from customs practiced by members of certain societies. The relationship that exists between heavy cigarette smokers and lung cancer now appears well established. A strong positive correlation has, moreover, been found to exist between the clay-pipe smokers in Ireland and cancer of the lip, while oral cancers are more prevalent among habitual snuff users than they are in the general population. A curious custom practiced by certain individuals in southern Asia, and known locally as chutta, is one that involves the smoking of cigars with the lighted end in their mouths. This practice has resulted in a high incidence of oral cancers. It is, moreover, a common practice among the natives of Kashmir to bind small charcoal-burning ovens around their waists during cold periods of the year to warm themselves. Cancers, which are known as Kangri burn cancers, commonly developed on the abdominal wall at points of irritation produced by the hot earthen oven. There are, furthermore, the betel nut chewers of south India who mix betel nuts with a cheap tobacco and finely crushed sea shells and it has been estimated that more than 75 percent of the oral cancers diagnosed in those regions were attributable to the persistent chewing of such a quid. This situation was aggravated further by the finding that diets of those individuals who developed cancers were seriously deficient in vitamin A, a vitamin that is known to promote keratinization in cells and that seems somehow to be involved in establishing resistance to the development of certain cancers. The importance of establishing a relationship between the occurrence of certain cancers and exposure to specific environmental influences including those present in the foods that we eat and water that we drink (254) is obvious. By application of such knowledge many cancers now arising in humans can be prevented.

Since man living in an urban industrial society is continually subjected to environmental carcinogens, studies of several different kinds are now underway in an attempt to find methods for preventing those cancer-producing agents from exerting their effects. Of the methods presently being tried and which appear to show promise when tested in experimental animals and in cultured tissues of animals is one which utilizes retinoids (255). These are compounds that are structurally related to vitamin A. The vitamin itself cannot safely be used because at the concentrations required to block the cancerous change in cells or to prevent cells from progressing from a precancerous to the cancerous state it is toxic and may cause liver damage. Some less toxic compounds of this type such as, for example, 13 bis retinoic acid appear to be more suitable and are now being tested for their abilities to prevent the cancerous change from being consummated in cells that have been exposed to environmental hazards. Such an approach, if found to be successful, would appear to be particularly applicable as preventative measures for those individuals who, because of their occupations, are exposed to higher than usual levels of carcinogenic substances. Controlled studies have now, in fact, been initiated to learn whether vitamin A-like compounds can inhibit the formation of certain cancers, particularly those of the bladder.

Although, as indicated above, certain chemical carcinogens have been shown to be cancer-producing without structural modifications, many others require structural changes in their molecules before their ultimate active form is realized. They must be activated enzymatically within a target cell so that they contain electron-deficient atoms (strong electrophiles) in their molecules which then react chemically with the electron-rich atoms (strong nucleophiles) found in the nucleic acids and proteins of a cell. Studies have been reported or are now underway either to attempt to prevent the conversion of such cancer-producing chemicals into their ultimate active forms or to trap the active form after it is produced in a target cell and thus render it harmless. It has been reported, for example, that 7,8-benzoflavone, which is an inhibitor of the enzyme aryl hydrocarbon hydroxylase (which converts carcinogenic hydrocarbons into their ultimate active forms), when applied to mouse skin together with the carcinogen 7,12-dimethylbenz[a]pyrene markedly retards the initiation of tumors (256). The cancer-producing N-2-fluorenylacetamide must, moreover, be converted to its strongly electrophilic sulfate ester by the cellular enzyme sulfotransferase to be effective in eliciting the formation of tumors. It has been found that a significant inhibition of liver tumors can be achieved in this instance by a depletion of the sulfate pool in cells of test organisms (257).

It has been suggested that, because of the necessity of having the ultimate active form of many carcinogens be strongly electrophilic, it might be possible to retard or inhibit the inception of tumors by flooding target cells with strong nucleophiles, thus trapping the active carcinogen before it binds to the critical macromolecules present in the cells. The results of some preliminary studies designed to test this hypothesis have shown that a partial inhibition of liver tumor initiation can, in fact, be achieved with the use of an excess of dietary amino acids such as methionine, cystine, or tryptophan (258). It has been proposed that such a mechanism may provide natural protection against the relatively small amounts of environmental carcinogens that are likely to be encountered at any particular time.

Certain antioxidants have, moreover, recently been found to decrease significantly cancer formation in mice and rats when administered just before or together with certain cancer-producing chemicals. It has been reported, for example, that sulfur-containing antioxidants such as dimethylthiocyanate, benzylthiocyanate or disulfiram, when incorporated into a diet for rats containing the chemical carcinogen 7,12-dimethylbenz[a]anthracene (which causes breast cancer when fed to female rats), the number of rats that developed these cancers as well as the number of cancers found per rat decreased markedly. Disulfiram was also found to inhibit significantly the development of cancers of the fore-stomach caused by benzo[a]pyrene in mice.

There are, moreover, differences that exist between normal cells and tumor cells that might be exploited therapeutically. One of these is concerned with differences in the method by which sugars are utilized. It was found many years ago that most but not all cancer cells break down sugars to lactic acid in the presence of oxygen and thus show what is known as aerobic glycolysis, while most but not all normal cells respire in the conventional manner (259). There have now been attempts to influence the respiratory behavior of tumor cells and thus to control tumor development. One of the more interesting examples of this is found in the case of the Plummer-Vinson syndrome which represents an early stage in the development of certain cancers of the esophagus and pharynx. It has been reported that if the diet of individuals suffering from this condition is heavily fortified with nicotinamide, flavin, and iron salts, which serve as coenzymes for the normal respiratory enzymes, the disease can not only be prevented but can, in some instances, be cured if the coenzymes are administered at an early enough time.

## CANCER DETECTION

If preventive measures fail and a cancer is initiated, it is imperative that a diagnosis of the new growth be made as early as possible and while it is still localized in its host. If localized cancers (equal to or less than one cubic centimeter in diameter) can be reached by the surgeon and/or by the radiotherapist, the probability of long term survival of the patient is estimated to be greater than 80 percent. It is, unfortunately, true that more than 60 percent of the cancer patients who are examined by physicians already have a disseminated disease by the time that a diagnosis is made. It is clearly desirable, therefore, to have an annual checkup by a competent internist, particularly after the age of 40. The American Cancer Society has, moreover, listed seven warning signals that should be looked for. They are:

Change in bowel or bladder habits

A sore that does not heal

Unusual bleeding or discharge

Thickening or lump in breast or elsewhere

CAUTION

Indigestion or difficulty in swallowing

Obvious change in wart or mole

Nagging cough or hoarseness

Radiology

The smallest tumor that is detectable by the more conventional methods of diagnosis such as palpation or X-ray examinations has a volume of one cubic centimeter and weighs about one gram. A tumor of that size may contain as many as one billion cancer cells. Methods for the detection of cancers when they are much smaller than that would, of course, be most desirable.

Diagnostic radiology has, nevertheless, played and is now playing a most important role not only in the detection of early, as yet asymptomatic cancers, but in evaluating the extent to which the disease has progressed in its host as well as in appraising the effectiveness of treatment of the disease. These methods, which include X-ray and fluoroscopic examinations, are particularly useful for examining hollow organs such as the lungs and gastrointestinal tract as well as air-filled spaces found in the nasal sinuses, larynx, bronchi of the lungs, etc. The familiar GI series and the barium enema are still among the most effective clinical methods for detecting cancers of the esophagus, stomach, and large intestine. Methods which now permit surgical sampling of tissue from a suspected new growth by means of a fluoroscopically controlled needle biopsy directly through the chest wall have, moreover, been developed. These methods extend the usefulness of chest radiography from a simple visualization of a tumor to the actual sampling of that tumor for diagnostic purposes.

### Mammography

One of the more significant recent advances for the visualization of early cancers involves the use of very low-dose X rays for the detection of breast cancers. This technique, which is known as mammography and of which several forms have been developed, has given encouraging results.

In 1972 the American Cancer Society and the National Cancer Institute jointly supported 27 National Breast Cancer Detection Clinics around the country. It was the purpose of those cancer detection centers to routinely screen approximately 270,000 women over the age of 35 for periods of up to ten years for possible cancers of the breast with the use of mammographic techniques. Among the approximately 130,000 women in the age group 35 to 50 that have now been screened at those diagnostic clinics, 308 cancers have been detected of which 137 or about 40 percent would have been missed had it not been for mammography. The detection rate in this age group is thus some 30 cancers for each 10,000 women screened. The question has recently been raised, therefore, whether repeated screening with the use of mammography can be justified in that age group when one considers the possible cell and tissue damage that may result from repeated annual exposures to even low doses of X-irradiation for periods of up to ten years. In women over 50, on the other hand, in which two-thirds of the breast cancer cases are found, the benefits of mammography are felt to outweigh the hazards that may result from repeated exposure to X-irradiation. Nevertheless, under new guidelines issued recently, the detection centers have now stopped routine mammographic screening of younger women unless those women are believed to face a higher than normal risk of developing breast cancer. Newer methods of mammography which are now being tested may overcome these difficulties. These precautionary measures are perhaps understandable in view of the unfortunate experience of some 40 years ago when X-irradiation was considered acceptable medical practice for the treatment of quite harmless but sometimes unsightly skin blemishes resulting from acne, a condition found most commonly in adolescents. Although this treatment for acne was often successful, multiple cancers of the face and neck as well as an increased incidence of thyroid cancers were found to occur in treated individuals in later years.

### Thermography

Another method that is now being developed for the detection of early asymptomatic cancers of the breast and elsewhere is known as thermography. It has long been recognized that abnormal conditions of many different kinds may cause the temperature at the surface of the affected organ to become slightly elevated. With the use of an instrument known as a thermographic camera the minutest changes in temperature at the surface of, for example, a breast can be readily detected. Thus very early cancers that may not be detectable by mammography or by physical examination are sometimes found with the use of this technique. Thermography has the advantage over mammography in that it can be used repeatedly as a diagnostic method without causing cell or tissue damage. However, thermography cannot be relied upon solely as a diagnostic tool because there are many factors such as infections, inflammation, and injury of various types that can upset the thermal equilibrium in tissues and organs.

## Endoscopic Examinations

Another very useful method for the detection of cancer in which significant progress has been made in recent years is one that involves endoscopic examination of the esophagus, stomach, and colon. With the use of this method excellent pictures can be taken of the internal surfaces of these structures and where a tumor is found biopsies and cytological washings of the tumor can be obtained in about 90 percent of the cases to confirm the diagnosis. There are, in addition, other specialized instruments that have proven useful for the early diagnosis of cancers. Among these might be mentioned the cystoscope for the detection of cancers of the bladder, the laparoscope for abdominal and pelvic malignancies and the colposcope for the diagnosis of cancers of the uterine cervix.

## Exfoliation Methods

This, then, brings us to another very useful technique, known as exfoliation, for the detection of early asymptomatic cancers. Normal cells that line the internal surfaces (and the external surfaces) of tissues and organs of the body are continually being sloughed off and if a cancer is present cancer cells may be found among the normal cells that are shed. Thus, cytological examination of the urine may reveal asymptomatic cancer of the urinary bladder or examination of sputum may provide evidence for cancer of the lung. Exfoliation techniques have also proved practical, particularly in Japan, for the early detection of cancer of the stomach. Doubtless, the most widely used and most successful mass screening application of these techniques has come from the Papanicolaou or Pap smears for the early detection of cancers of many types but especially of the uterine cervix. On a world-wide basis they are the most prevalent cancers in women and in the United States they are second only to breast cancers. The widespread use of this method for the early detection of cancer of the cervix has now led to many cures that would otherwise not have been possible.

### Other Methods for Cancer Detection

Other methods for the detection of select cancers depend upon the release into the urine or the serum of specific hormones, enzymes, or antigens. These include, for example, specific tests of urine for the presence of chorionic gonadotrophin which is characteristic of choriocarcinomas, or acid phosphatase in the case of carcinomas of the prostate.

There are, in addition, the so-called embryonic or fetal antigens which are secreted by cancer cells and may be present in the blood of individuals having particular types of cancer (260). The first of these is the carcinoembryonic antigen which is often found in patients with cancer of the colon, rectum, pancreas, and certain other organs. This antigen may sometimes be found in the absence of tumors, particularly in the case of inflammatory reactions or regenerative conditions. A second antigen, the so-called alpha fetoprotein, is often present in blood of patients with liver tumors (hepatomas) or with embryonal carcinomas, while a third antigen is a fetal gastric sulphoglycoprotein which is found in the gastric juice not only in 96 percent of patients with gastric carcinomas but in about 14 percent of patients with gastric ulcers as well. All three types of antigen are found in normal embryonic or fetal tissues but are not commonly found in most adult normal tissues. Studies are now being carried out to learn whether these antigens can be made to serve as useful diagnostic tools for the presence of otherwise undetectable cancers.

There are other promising methods that are now in the early stages of development and that may ultimately prove useful for the detection of early cancers. One of these is known as the leukocyte adherence inhibition method. This test measures the decrease in the capacity of white blood cells to adhere to glass surfaces following incubation with soluble extracts of specific tumors of different kinds (261).

Another method that is now being studied for the detection of early cancers of several different kinds is the so-called "T" or thymus lymphocyte rosette test. It has long been known that "T" lymphocytes possess the peculiar ability of clustering normal red blood cells around their surface in rosette fashion. This observation has now been found to be useful for the detection of certain early cancers and a decrease in the ability of the "T" lymphocytes to form rosettes is taken to be an early warning sign of the possible presence of cancer (262).

## CANCER TREATMENT

### Surgery

Once a cancer has been detected it is imperative that it be dealt with at the earliest possible time. Surgical procedures are at present the most widely used and most successful form of cancer therapy. To cure a cancer by means of surgery the new growth must, however, be removed while it is still localized in its host since once it has spread it has gone beyond the reach of successful surgery. If, nevertheless, an early diagnosis is made and prompt and competent surgery is performed, the rate of cure of many different kinds of cancers can be increased significantly.

In addition to curative surgery, preventative surgery involving the timely removal of precancerous or other suspect but not yet cancerous lesions is now being routinely practiced in certain quarters as a prophylactic measure. Doubtless many growths that would ultimately develop into cancers are eliminated by such preventative measures.

With the recent development of surgical techniques for the successful transplantation of normal organs, new methods for cancer control may be realized and the replacement of a vital organ seriously damaged by cancer has already been achieved in a few instances. As these techniques are perfected certain of the most serious cancers may eventually be dealt with successfully.

Finally, the surgeon can and does provide a most useful service to patients whose cancers have progressed beyond the point where they can be successfully dealt with by any method. In such instances the surgeon is often called upon to apply palliative surgical procedures to alleviate pain and suffering and thus bring comfort to a patient during the terminal phase of his or her illness.

## Radiation Therapy

Methods that are second only to surgery as a means for the curative or palliative treatment of many different kinds of cancers are those that make use of ionizing radiations such as X rays, gamma rays from radioactive cobalt 60, and electrons. Ionizing radiations are believed to exert their deleterious effects on cells by causing both single- and double-stranded breaks that account for the lethal effects of the radiation. Radiation therapy has made enormous strides during the past quarter-century due largely to the development of highly sophisticated and versatile machines that produce beams in the multimillion electron volt energy range. Such beams are often effective against deep-seated cancers of many kinds that could not easily be reached with the lower voltage instruments previously used. It is estimated that currently radiation therapy is used in more than one-half of all cancer cases at one stage or another during the development of the new growth. Comparative five-year survival rates of patients with different kinds of cancers attest to the efficacy of radiation therapy carried out with the use of the newer megavolt machines. While the bulk of many cancers may, in effect, melt away under the influence of ionizing radiation, there are often recurrences of the same cancer. This may, in part at least, be attributable to the fact that cells are about three times more sensitive to radiation damage in the presence of oxygen than in its absence. The cells of many cancers outgrow their blood supply and such cells survive in the absence of adequate oxygen. The recurrence of many cancers after an initially good radiotherapeutic response has been attributed, in some instances at least, to a regrowth of such cells.

Certain other nuclear particles, notably neutrons and negative pi mesons, are now under study as possible substitutes for X rays and electrons. These particles are much less dependent on oxygen for their effects and in the case of pi mesons a much more precise and selective localization of the beam energy to the area occupied by the cancer is possible than with the other forms of radiation.

### Tumor Angiogenesis Factor

Since surgery and/or radiation therapy are now quite effective in dealing with many early cancers that have remained localized in their hosts, a most important area for study would appear to be concerned with the development of methods for keeping cancers localized and thus preventing their dissemination throughout a host. One such method now being investigated is based on the knowledge that many cancers require an adequate blood supply for their continued growth and if deprived of a blood supply they remain small and localized in their hosts. It has now been found that many if not all solid cancers produce a specific substance which diffuses from the cancer cells and which, when applied to appropriate normal test systems (chorioallantoic membranes of nine- to ten-day-old chick embryos or the cornea of a rabbit's eye), induces in a few days the formation of an intricate network of normal blood capillaries in those tissues (263). This capillary-inducing substance, which is known as the tumor angiogenesis factor, has not at the time of this writing been characterized chemically. Thus, cells of many cancers ensure not only their own survival but their continued growth by virtue of their ability to synthesize the tumor angiogenesis factor. This, then, is a most important control point in the development of many cancers. If ways could be found either to neutralize the capillary-inducing effects of the tumor angiogenesis factor or to inhibit the formation of capillaries in the presence of that factor, an important step forward would have been taken. It has now been reported (264) that there is a diffusible substance present in normal cartilage obtained from several species of animals that can largely prevent the formation of capillaries induced by the tumor angiogenesis factor. The precise nature of this diffusible factor and its mode of action in preventing the formation of capillaries has not as yet been entirely resolved (see Fig. 28).

A second approach that is now being actively investigated in the laboratory is one involving the use of specific chemicals which have been found in animal experimentation studies

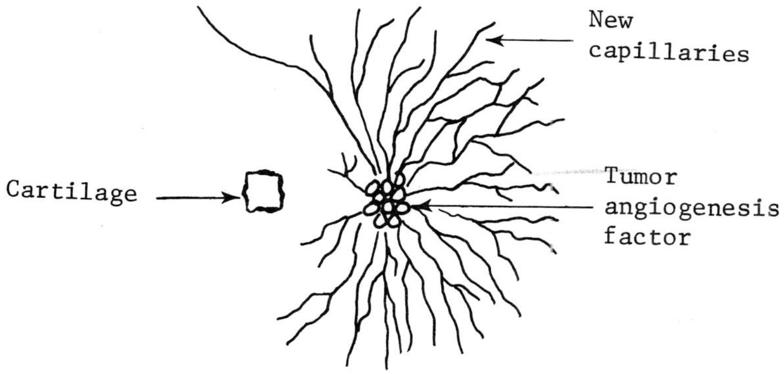


FIGURE 28. An experiment of the type which illustrates that malignant cells produce a substance, the tumor angiogenesis factor, which encourages the formation of new blood vessels in normal host tissues. These new blood vessels provide the cancer cells with nutrients and oxygen and remove metabolic wastes from the tumor; without them the cancers could not survive, at least not in large masses. In the above experiment a small amount of the tumor angiogenesis factor was placed on the chorioallantoic membrane of a chick embryo and many new blood capillaries developed. It was reported, further, that capillary formation could be largely inhibited by an as yet uncharacterized but diffusible substance present in cartilage.

to be more effective in preventing metastases than in inhibiting the growth of the primary tumor.

### Chemotherapy

Unlike surgery and radiation therapy, the use of anticancer drugs makes possible the treatment of disseminated as well as localized cancers. Several distinct classes of anticancer drugs are now being ~~used~~ therapeutically. These include alkylating agents which arrest ~~cell~~ growth by cross-linking reactive groups in the chromosomal DNA and thus render that molecule incapable of replicating. Some of the most commonly used alkylating agents are the nitrogen mustards which were largely developed during the Second World War in a search for more effective vesicant war gases. Certain of these alkylating agents such as myleran, mustargen, and leukeran have been used for the treatment of leukemias and lymphomas while others such as melphalan, thiotepa, and cyclophosphamide are, in addition, used to treat solid cancers of several different types. A second group of compounds being successfully used as anticancer agents are the antimetabolites. These substances are structural analogues of vitamins, amino acids, purines or pyrimidines, or other essential metabolites. The antimetabolites compete with essential metabolites for active sites on the surface of specific enzymes and prevent the normal synthesis or utilization of the essential metabolite by a cell. This, in turn, interferes with normal growth processes by inhibiting cell division. Some of the most commonly used anticancer antimetabolites are folic acid antagonists and methotrexate is an excellent example of such an antagonist that has been used either by itself or, more commonly, in combination with other anticancer drugs for the treatment of a wide variety of tumors including, among others, choriocarcinomas, a highly malignant cancer that arises from the placenta, cancers of the head, neck, and cervix, as well as acute leukemias. Other antimetabolites that are being used usually in combination with other drugs are 5-fluorouracil for cancers of the breast, large intestine, and certain ovarian tumors, cytarabine hydrochloride and 6-thioguanine for some of the leukemias, and 6-mercaptopurine for certain types of acute and chronic leukemias.

A third group of anticancer chemicals are the antibiotics, certain members of which have been so dramatically effective for the treatment of bacterial diseases of many kinds. One of the most widely used of these for the treatment of lymphomas, breast, thyroid, bronchiogenic carcinomas, as well as sarcomas of several types is adriamycin. Other antibiotics being used are bleomycin for the treatment of lymphomas, squamous cell carcinomas, and testicular carcinomas, and dactinomycin for testicular carcinomas, Wilms's tumor, rhabdomyosarcoma, osteogenic and certain other sarcomas.

Examples of a fourth group of anticancer chemicals, which are naturally occurring plant products, are the *Vinca* alkaloids, vinblastine sulfate and vincristine sulfate. These substances arrest cell division by interfering with the formation of the mitotic spindle during metaphase in the cell cycle. The former has been used for the treatment of Hodgkin's disease and other lymphomas while vincristine sulfate has, in addition, been shown to be effective for the treatment of acute lymphocytic leukemia. What appears to be a promising new anticancer drug and which has been given the trivial designation PS-K was isolated from a common mushroom species known as Kawaradake in Japan and has been reported to be effective against stomach cancer, lung cancers, and cancer of the intestine. PS-K is said to produce no harmful side effects and is believed to exert its beneficial effects by enhancing the immune response of the patient.

Finally, certain hormone-dependent cancers such as breast and prostatic carcinomas are susceptible to hormonal manipulation and may be treated effectively in this way. While certain cancers such as the choriocarcinomas and osteosarcomas (methotrexate) as well as Burkitt's lymphoma (cyclophosphamide) have been successfully treated with single drugs, the inability to treat many advanced cancers in this way has led to the use of multidrug therapy. The theory behind the use of multidrug therapy rests on the following principles (265): (1) the different drugs should exert their deleterious effects on the growth of cancer cells by different mechanisms; (2) each drug should be administered during the stage in the cell cycle when it will exert its maximum effects; (3) the type of toxicities shown by the drugs used should be different so that each drug can be given at its maximum dose; and (4) each drug used in the combination should show activity against the specific tumor that is being treated.

The effectiveness of multidrug therapy based on the principles listed above is dramatically illustrated in the case of Hodgkin's disease. In this instance four drugs, the alkylating agent mustargen, the plant alkaloid vincristine, the synthetic chemical procarbazine hydrochloride and prednisone, which is used in hormone-dependent cancer therapy, when applied in combination against advanced Hodgkin's disease have been found to result in a high number of remissions in this form of cancer. Multiple drug therapy has also been found to be effective against acute lymphocytic leukemias, testicular carcinomas, and non-Hodgkin's lymphomas such as reticulum cell sarcomas and lymphosarcomas.

More commonly, however, single and multiple drug therapy is used in combination with and following surgery and radiation therapy. Improvement in the treatment of breast cancer has recently been claimed by using a combination of three drugs, methotrexate, 5-fluorouracil, and cyclophosphamide, following surgery in those women whose cancers had spread to the lymph nodes prior to the surgical removal of the cancer from the breast. Many of these women were alive for more than two years after the treatment began (266).

The basic premise on which chemotherapy is based is that cancer cells differ in some exploitable way from normal cells. Unfortunately, no one has yet discovered specific qualitative differences that can be exploited therapeutically in the generality of cancers. Most effective anticancer drugs affect growth processes generally and, since many normal cells grow and divide at rates that approach or even exceed those of many cancer cells, the normal cells are also affected by the drug. This leads to toxicity and at times great discomfort to patients being treated with anticancer drugs. In some instances the toxic effects due to an anticancer drug such as methotrexate may be decreased by leucovorin or the citrovorum factor if treatment is begun at the first signs of toxicity. In many other instances it is not as yet possible to alleviate the toxicity of the drugs. Yet an estimated eight percent of all early cancers can now be cured with the use of anticancer drug therapy and this figure attests to the usefulness of this approach for the control of cancer.

The ideal anticancer drug would be one that would selectively destroy or normalize cancer cells while doing little or no damage to normal cells. We have alluded to one such substance earlier which is naturally occurring and nontoxic and which causes acute myelocytic leukemic cells of humans in culture to mature and differentiate into granulocytes and macrophages which have lost their malignant properties.

An example in which differences between normal cells and tumor cells can be exploited therapeutically is found in the case of certain leukemias and lymphosarcomas, the cells of which possess an absolute exogenous requirement for the amino acid L-asparagine for their growth. Most normal cells are able to synthesize that compound and do not require an exogenous source of it for growth. It was found that by introducing into the bloodstream of leukemic patients the enzyme L-asparaginase, which destroys the free asparagine in the blood, dramatic remissions were obtained in patients with L-asparagine-dependent leukemias (267). In many instances, however, some leukemic cells remained that did not share this asparagine-dependence and as those cells multiplied this form of therapy became inadequate. This system, nevertheless, represents a model and if other differences between normal and tumor cells can be identified that are closer to the mechanisms underlying the heritable cellular change than is asparagine-dependence, they may perhaps be more profitably exploited therapeutically.

## Interferons

There are a number of different types of naturally occurring nontoxic substances that are now being actively studied as potential anticancer agents. One of these classes of substances, the interferons, has been found in animal tests to have profound effects not only in preventing the inception and retarding the spread of certain leukemias and solid tumors but in arresting progressions as well as in causing regressions of advanced tumors in mice. The interferons, which are small protein molecules, were initially found to be produced by and to be released from cells infected with a virus. These substances diffuse to neighboring cells and protect those cells not only from the virus initially involved in the infection but from a wide spectrum of other viruses as well. It is now believed that many viral infections generally are held in check as a result of this special defense mechanism. The interferons are produced in many animal species that range from the lower vertebrates to man. Interferon-like substances have also been found in cells of higher plants following viral infection. These substances have also been found to be species-specific in the sense that they are optimally active in cells of the species that produce them.

The antitumor effects of the interferons may clearly operate through mechanisms other than those involved in inhibiting the replication of oncogenic viruses and these may include inhibition of tumor cell division, modulation of lymphocyte function, enhancement of the phagocytic activity of the macrophages, and perhaps also to modify other components of the immune system particularly the serum complement levels (268, 269).

Studies on the use of interferons as anticancer agents in man have been seriously hampered in the past by an inability to obtain sufficient amounts of them for extensive clinical trials. Methods have now been developed for the large scale continuous production of high titer interferon preparations and these methods should soon yield amounts sufficient for purification, chemical characterization, and perhaps synthesis of these substances for more extensive clinical trials in humans than have been possible up to the present.

Chalones

A second group of naturally occurring nontoxic substances that are being investigated as possible anticancer agents are collectively known as chalones. These substances appear to be importantly involved not only in the regulation of the cell division process but in cellular differentiation as well. The chalones are tissue-specific compounds which inhibit cell division and which are synthesized by and have been isolated from such diverse cell types as epidermal cells, liver and kidney cells, granulocytes, as well as from a number of other different and distinct cell types (270). The chalones are, moreover, not a homogeneous class of compounds but differ significantly from one another. The liver chalone (271) and the mammary cell chalone (272), for example, have been found to be of low molecular weight, while the epidermal chalone is a basic glycoprotein having a molecular weight of about 35,000 (273). The epidermal chalone is effective in blocking cell division only in the presence of adrenalin. Since the antimitotic effect of these substances is tissue-specific and since they are essentially nontoxic, they would appear to represent an almost ideal group of substances for use in the suppression of growth of those tumors that have lost an ability to synthesize their own chalones but remain sensitive to the inhibitory effects of those substances. Although some success has been claimed in arresting the growth of certain tumors (274-276a), a great deal more work will have to be done before an evaluation of the effectiveness of chalones can be made.

### Immunological Approaches to Control

An important difference between normal cells and tumor cells that is now being exploited therapeutically is found in the new antigens that are often present at the surface of tumor cells. These new tumor antigens are different from those found at the surface of normal cells and are therefore recognized by the immune system of an animal as being foreign and, hence, elicit specific immune responses against them. The tumor antigens may be detected in a variety of ways and one of the most direct of these is the demonstration that inbred strains of mice that have, for example, been immunized against antigens present in a specific tumor will often reject implants of that same tumor. Although the evidence for tumor immunity in humans is more indirect, there is, nevertheless, considerable evidence available to show that immune responses may keep early tumors in check and may even cause spontaneous regressions of certain advanced cancers. The important role that the immune response may play in the control of cancer in humans is evidenced not only by the finding that individuals with primary immunodeficiency diseases such as the Wiskott-Aldrich syndrome, IgA deficiency, and sex-linked agammaglobulinemia, etc., have a significantly greater than normal risk of developing cancer, but individuals who are treated over extended periods of time with immunosuppressant drugs also have a greater than normal risk of developing cancers.

There are several different kinds of white blood cells that are importantly involved in protecting higher animals from what the organism recognizes as being a foreign substance. There are the plasma cells which produce specific antibodies against foreign proteins and certain other complex molecules. These antibodies are released from the plasma cells and circulate freely in the blood stream and other body fluids. This is known as humoral immunity. There are, in addition, the cell-mediated immune responses which are carried out by essentially three different types of white blood cells. The polymorphonuclear leukocytes engulf and often destroy foreign invaders such as disease-producing bacteria. This type of white blood cell does not appear to play a role in the development of immunity to cancer. There are, in addition, the lymphocytes and the large scavenger cells known as the macrophages which together constitute the major immune defense mechanism against cancer cells. There are two different classes of lymphocytes which are known as T (thymus) lymphocytes and B (bursa) lymphocytes. The B type cells interact with foreign antigens and synthesize and secrete into the blood stream specific antibodies to those antigens. The T lymphocytes, on the other hand, also synthesize specific antibody-like compounds but these substances remain localized at the surface of the T cells. It is by means of these surface antibodies that the T lymphocytes recognize the tumor-specific transplantation antigens. Upon recognition, the T cells release substances that initiate a series of complex reactions between T cells, B cells, and macrophages that may ultimately result in the destruction of the cancer cells. Cancers are often found to be infiltrated with large numbers of T lymphocytes. Lymphocytes from patients with certain cancers have been found, moreover, to inhibit *in vitro* growth of not only the patient's tumor cells but also tumor cells of patients with the same disease (277).

The T lymphocytes, upon making contact with cancer cells, release a specific substance(s) which attracts macrophages to the site of the tumor where they may aid in its destruction. The macrophages recognize cancer cells through what has come to be known as the recognition factor. This substance appears to be an alpha globulin and may be present in the blood of cancer patients. An inverse relationship has been found to exist between the amount of recognition factor present in the blood stream and the extent to which a cancer has developed in a host. It is believed that a complexing of the macrophage recognition factor with tumor cells is the first step required for the destruction of those cells by the macrophages. The failure of the recognition factor-synthesizing system would, on the other hand, permit tumor cells to go unrecognized by the macrophages and thus escape destruction by those cells.

It thus appears that both humoral and, most importantly, cellular immune responses are involved in the development of immunity to cancer cells not only in animals but in humans as well.

Reasons for failure of the immune system. The question that might now reasonably be asked is why, if cancer cells are antigenic and are recognized by a host as foreign objects, are they not completely destroyed by the immune response of a host? There are very good reasons for this and any one of a number of factors that suppress the normal immune response could and doubtless do play an important role in determining whether a given tumor will be affected.

One of the more important of these is the finding that

there may be blocking factors present in the blood of cancer patients that protect the cancer cells from the T-lymphocyte-mediated immune response. These blocking factors are believed to act by preventing the recognition of the cancer cells by the T-lymphocytes. The production of these blocking factors appears, in most instances, to require the continuous presence of the tumor antigens and are oftentimes lost when the tumor is removed or otherwise destroyed. Although the exact nature of these blocking molecules is not known, they are felt to be antibodies or antigen-antibody complexes (277). That such blocking factors may exist in sera of tumor-bearing animals is evidenced from the following type of experiment. It has been reported that sera of tumor-bearing animals are capable of inhibiting the specific T-lymphocyte immune response to the tumor-specific antigen _in vitro_. It was found, however, that when the T-lymphocytes are isolated from the blood of such animals and freed of serum they are capable of killing the tumor cells _in vitro_. When that serum was again added back to the experimental test system, the killing effect of the T-lymphocytes on the tumor cells was blocked. It is clear, therefore, that some factor or factors present in sera of tumor-bearing animals inhibit the cytotoxic effect that the lymphocytes exert on the tumor cells _in vitro_. It now appears that essentially three types of blocking substances may be found in serum of tumor-bearing animals. These are, first, the tumor-derived antigens that are found circulating freely in the blood of tumor-bearing animals. These tumor antigens can, in some instances at least, block the tumor-destroying activity of the T-lymphocytes when mixed with them. The transplantation antigens have, on the other hand, no detectable blocking activity when they remain present at the surface of the tumor cells. A second blocking factor present in sera of tumor-bearing animals are the tumor-specific antibodies. These antibodies can block the T-lymphocyte-mediated immune response at the tumor-cell level. Finally, a mixture of tumor-derived antigens and the specific antibodies can block the immune response at both the T-lymphocyte and tumor-cell levels.

It has been found possible to again unblock the inhibitory effect of serum from tumor-bearing animals by treating such sera with the specific antibodies which neutralize the effects of those tumor antigens and antigen-antibody complexes and which are responsible for the blocking reactions. Substances with unblocking properties may ultimately provide a useful immunological approach for the prevention of tumor formation as well as for the treatment of existing tumors. Other immunosuppressive substances derived from tumor cells have been described (278).

There are other reasons why the immune system of a host may fail. One of these involves immunoselection. As in any dividing population of cells, as a tumor grows the cells that comprise the new growth often differ from one another and some of the cells are more antigenic than others. It is the least antigenic cells that would be expected to survive and such a selection process could well account for the poor antigenicity shown by cells of many advanced cancers. The inadequacy of the immune response in a host to cancer cells may be demonstrated in other ways. It has been found that when a massive, rapidly growing cancer that has developed in a host is removed surgically, the animal often resists reimplantation of its own cancer cells, indicating that the immune system is, in fact, functional but that that system is simply overwhelmed by too great a challenge from the developing cancer. Finally, the immune system may fail because of a phenomenon known as immunological tolerance which is found to occur when an animal is exposed to an antigen very early in life before the immune system has developed fully. This phenomenon is well illustrated in the case of certain vertically transmitted viruses in which the animal in later life is tolerant to those viruses, and even when large amounts of fully antigenic virus particles are injected into such animals antibodies do not form and the animals are thus incapable of immune defense against them.

It has been observed, moreover, that immune white blood cells may actually stimulate the growth of cancer cells when present in small numbers while inhibiting their growth when present in large numbers (279).

Immunoadjuvants. Despite these problems, tumor immunology offers a promising approach for the control of cancer particularly when used in association with other forms of therapy. Methods are now being sought to increase the immunogenicity of cancer cells and thus make them more vulnerable to attack by the immune system, as well as to increase the immune response of the host with the use of immunoadjuvants. The immunoadjuvants most commonly used are of a nonspecific type involving bacteria or bacterial or fungal extracts. BCG, which is an attenuated form of the tubercle bacillus (280-282), and *Corynebacterium parvum* (283), which is related to the diphtheria-causing bacterium, have been used clinically as immunoadjuvants against cancers of several types and some dramatic remissions have been reported in some instances. The efficacy and safety of these agents as well as other immunostimulants such as Coley's toxin or the antihelminthic leucumisole remain to be established (284). The mechanisms by which these nonspecific immunoadjuvants stimulate local and general immunological responses is as yet poorly understood, and the entire problem of immune enhancement is clearly an important area for further study.

Cancer vaccines. Although vaccines prepared with the use of a patient's own cancer cells have long been used with questionable results for the control of cancer, very recent studies from Hawaii and from Canada have claimed success in preventing the recurrence of cancers of the stomach and lungs, respectively. Although such preliminary trials appear promising, claims of success with such vaccines have been limited and more extensive clinical studies are clearly needed to accurately assess their efficacy and toxicity.

## OUTLOOK FOR THE FUTURE

This, then, is a brief overview of the multifaceted world-wide attack that is now being carried out in the battle against cancer. There seems little doubt that enormous progress has been made during the past few decades not only in our understanding of cancer as a basic biological phenomenon but in dealing with it as a major public health problem as well. While the difficulties in dealing in a practical way with this very complex disease must certainly never be underestimated, sufficient progress has now been made in our understanding of the causes of cancer that if we are prepared to apply that knowledge to our everyday lives the incidence of cancer can doubtless be markedly reduced. Encouraging, too, are the technical advances that have been made and that are now being made for the detection of early cancers as well as for the treatment of certain cancers. Some (for example, choriocarcinomas), which only a few short years ago were invariably fatal unless dealt with very early, can now be cured in 75 percent of patients with combination chemotherapy even when this cancer has become widely disseminated. Certain other more commonly found cancers, including those of the breast, now appear to be responding favorably to the therapeutic measures being applied to them. As new knowledge becomes available, further progress in dealing with cancer effectively can reasonably be expected. While much more clearly needs to be done, there now appears reason for optimism especially over the longer term.

## REFERENCES


1. Oberling, C. The Riddle of Cancer. Translated by W. H. Woglom. 196 pp. Yale University Press, New Haven, 1944.
2. Pott, P. Chirurgical Observations Relative to the Cataract, the Polypus of the Nose, the Cancer of the Scrotum, the Different Kinds of Ruptures, and the Mortification of the Toes and Feet. 208 pp. Hawes, London, 1775.
3. Bichat, [M. F.] X. Anatomie Générale, Appliquée à la Physiologie et à la Médecine. Nouvelle éd. 4 Vols. J. A. Brosson et J. S. Chaudé, Paris, 1821.
4. Schwann, T. Mikroskopische Untersuchungen über die Uebereinstimmung in der Struktur und dem Wachsthum der Thiere und Pflanzen. 270 pp. G. E. Reimer, Berlin, 1839.
5. Müller, J. Ueber den feineren Bau und die Formen der krankhaften Geschwülste. Lief. 1. G. Reimer, Berlin, 1838.
6. Virchow, R. Die krankhaften Geschwülste. p. 89. A. Hirschwald, Berlin, 1863.
7. Cohnheim, J. F. Vorlesungen über allgemeine Pathologie. 1:622-691. A. Hirschwald, Berlin, 1877.
8. Hanau, A. N. Experimentelle Uebertragung von Carcinom von Ratte auf Ratte. Arch. Klin. Chir. 39:678-679. 1889.
9. Wehr. Weitere Mittheilungen über die positiven Ergebnisse von Carcinom-Ueberimpfungen von Hund auf Hund. Arch. Klin. Chir. 39:226-228. 1889.
10. Loeb, L. On transplantation of tumors. J. Med. Res. n.s. 1:28-38. 1901.

11. Jensen, C. O. Nogle forsøg med kraeftsvulster. (af lektor, 1901.) Hospitalstidende, 4 R, 10:489-502. 1902.
12. Jensen, C. O. Experimentelle Untersuchungen über Krebs bei Mäusen. Zentralbl. Bakteriol. Parasitenk., Abt. I, Orig. 34:28-34, 122-143. 1903.
13. Jensen, C. O. Von echten Geschwülsten bei Pflanzen. Deuxième Conférence Internationale pour l'Etude du Cancer, Paris, 1910. Rapport (F. Alcan, ed.) p. 243-254. Paris, 1911. (Reprinted as: Medd. Kgl. Vet.- og Landbohøjskoles Serumlab. VII.)
14. Boveri, T. The Origin of Malignant Tumors. Translated by M. Boveri. 119 pp. Williams and Wilkins, Baltimore, 1929.
15. Smith, E. F., and Townsend, C. O. A plant-tumor of bacterial origin. Science 25:671-673. 1907.
16. Ellermann, V., and Bang, O. Experimentelle Leukämie bei Hühnern. Zentralbl. Bakteriol. Parasitenk., Abt. I, Orig. 46:595-609. 1908.
17. Rous, P. A transmissible avian neoplasm. (Sarcoma of the common fowl.) J. Exptl. Med. 12:696-705. 1910.
18. Andrewes, C. H. Viruses in relation to the aetiology of tumours. Lancet II:63-69, 117-124. 1934.
19. Marie, P., Clunet, J., and Raulot-Lapointe, G. Contribution à l'étude du développement des tumeurs malignes sur les ulcères de roentgen. Bull. Assoc. Franç. Etude Cancer 3:404-426. 1910.
20. Marie, P., Clunet, J., and Raulot-Lapointe, G. Hérédité des caractères acquis, chez les cellules néoplasiques. Bull. Assoc. Franç. Etude Cancer 3:166-172. 1911.
21. Marie, P., Clunet, J., and Raulot-Lapointe, G. Nouveau cas de tumeur maligne provoquée par une radiodermite expérimentale chez le rat blanc. Bull. Assoc. Franc. Etude Cancer 5:125-135. 1912.
22. Rehn, L. Blasengeschwülste bei Fuchsin-Arbeitern. Arch. Klin. Chir. 50:588-600. 1895.
23. Yamagiwa, K., and Ichikawa, K. Experimental study of the pathogenesis of carcinoma. J. Cancer Res. 3:1-29. 1918.
24. Cook, J. W., Hewett, C. L., and Hieger, I. The isolation of a cancer-producing hydrocarbon from coal tar. Pts. I, II, and III. J. Chem. Soc. 1933:395-405. 1933.
25. Wieland, H., and Dane, E. Untersuchungen über die Konstitution der Gallensäuren. LII. Mitt. Über die Haftstelle der Seitenkette. Z. Physiol. Chem. 219:240-244. 1933.
26. Black, H. S., and Douglas, D. R. A model system for the evaluation of the role of cholesterol α-oxide in ultraviolet carcinogenesis. Cancer Res. 32:2630-2632. 1972.

27. Maugh, T. H., II. Chemical carcinogenesis: a long-neglected field blossoms. Science 183:940-944. 1974.
28. Slye, M. The incidence and inheritability of spontaneous cancer in mice. (Preliminary report) Z. Krebsforsch. 13:500-504. 1913.
29. Slye, M. The incidence and inheritability of spontaneous tumors in mice. (Second report) J. Med. Res. 30 (n.s. 25):281-298. 1914.
30. Muller, H. J. Artificial transmutation of the gene. Science 66:84-87. 1927.
31. Beadle, G. W., and Tatum, E. L. Genetic control of biochemical reactions in Neurospora. Proc. Natl. Acad. Sci. USA 27:499-506. 1941.
32. Avery, O. T., MacLeod, C. M., and McCarty, M. Studies on the chemical nature of the substance inducing transformation of pneumococcal types. J. Exptl. Med. 79:137-158. 1944.
33. Griffith, F. The significance of pneumococcal types. J. Hygiene 27:113-159. 1928.
34. Chargaff, E. Chemical specificity of nucleic acids and mechanism of their enzymatic degradation. Experientia 6:201-209. 1950.
35. Wilkins, M. H. F., Stokes, A. R., and Wilson, H. R. Molecular structure of deoxypentose nucleic acids. Nature 171:738-740. 1953.
36. Franklin, R. E., and Gosling, R. G. Molecular configuration in sodium thymonucleate. Nature 171:740-741. 1953.
37. Watson, J. D., and Crick, F. H. C. A structure for deoxyribose nucleic acid. Nature 171:737-738. 1953.
38. Watson, J. D., and Crick, F. H. C. Genetical implications of the structure of deoxyribonucleic acid. Nature 171:964-967. 1953.
39. Khorana, H. G., Agarwal, K. L., Besmer, P., et al. Total synthesis of the structural gene for the precursor of a tyrosine suppressor transfer RNA from Escherichia coli. 1. General introduction. J. Biol. Chem. 251:565-570. 1976.
40. Crick, F. H. C., Barnett, L., Brenner, S., et al. General nature of the genetic code for proteins. Nature 192:1227-1232. 1961.
41. Nirenberg, M. W. The genetic code: II. Scient. Am. 208 (No. 3):80-86, 89-91, 93-94. 1963.
42. Mirsky, A. E., and Ris, H. Variable and constant components of chromosomes. Nature 163:666-667. 1949.
43. Vendrely, R., and Vendrely, C. La teneur du noyau cellulaire en acide désoxyribonucléique à travers les organes, les individus et les espèces animales.

Experientia 4:434-436. 1948.
44. Vasil, V., and Hildebrandt, A. C. Differentiation of tobacco plants from single, isolated cells in microcultures. Science 150:889-892. 1965.
45. Steward, F. C., Mapes, M. O., Kent, A. E., et al. Growth and development of cultured plant cells. Science 143: 20-27. 1964.
46. Gurdon, J. B., and Uehlinger, V. "Fertile" intestine nuclei. Nature 210:1240-1241. 1966.
47. Painter, T. S. A new method for the study of chromosome rearrangements and the plotting of chromosome maps. Science 78:585-586. 1933.
48. Painter, T. S. Salivary chromosomes and the attack on the gene. J. Heredity 25:465-476. 1934.
49. Bridges, C. B. Salivary chromosome maps. J. Heredity 26:60-64. 1935.
50. Beermann, W. Ein Balbiani-Ring als Locus einer Speicheldrüsen-Mutation. Chromosoma 12:1-25. 1961.
51. Jacob, F., and Monod, J. Genetic regulatory mechanisms in the synthesis of proteins. J. Mol. Biol. 3:318-356. 1961.
52. Hamperl, H. Ueber die Entwicklung ("Progression") von Tumoren. Wien. Klin. Wchnschr. 69:201-205. 1957.
53. Berenblum, I. The mechanism of carcinogenesis. A study of the significance of cocarcinogenic action and related phenomena. Cancer Res. 1:807-814. 1941.
54. Rous, P., and Kidd, J. G. Conditional neoplasms and subthreshold neoplastic states. A study of the tar tumors of rabbits. J. Exptl. Med. 73:365-390. 1941.
55. MacKenzie, I., and Rous, P. The experimental disclosure of latent neoplastic changes in tarred skin. J. Exptl. Med. 73:391-416. 1941.
56. de Terra, N. Macronuclear DNA synthesis in Stentor: regulation by a cytoplasmic initiator. Proc. Natl. Acad. Sci. USA 57:607-614. 1967.
57. Prescott, D. M., and Goldstein, L. Nuclear-cytoplasmic interaction in DNA synthesis. Science 155:469-470. 1967.
58. Graham, C. F., Arms, K., and Gurdon, J. B. The induction of DNA synthesis by frog egg cytoplasm. Develop. Biol. 14:349-381. 1966.
59. Gurdon, J. B. On the origin and persistence of a cytoplasmic state inducing nuclear DNA synthesis in frogs' eggs. Proc. Natl. Acad. Sci. USA 58:545-552. 1967.
60. Gelfant, S. A new theory on the mechanism of cell division. Symp. Intern. Soc. Cell Biol. 2:229-259. 1963.

61. Braun, A. C., Guest Ed. Plant Tumor Research. 235 pp. (Progr. Exptl. Tumor Res., 15) Karger, Basel, 1972.
62. Jazwinski, S. M., Wang, J. L., and Edelman, G. M. Initiation of replication in chromosomal DNA induced by extracts from proliferating cells. Proc. Natl. Acad. Sci. USA 73:2231-2235. 1976.
63. Shodell, M. Environmental stimuli in the progression of BHK/21 cells through the cell cycle. Proc. Natl. Acad. Sci. USA 69:1455-1459. 1972.
64. Braun, A. C. The activation of two growth-substance systems accompanying the conversion of normal to tumor cells in crown gall. Cancer Res. 16:53-56. 1956.
65. Braun, A. C. A physiological basis for autonomous growth of the crown-gall tumor cell. Proc. Natl. Acad. Sci. USA 44:344-349. 1958.
66. Braun, A. C. Thermal studies on the factors responsible for tumor initiation in crown gall. Am. J. Botany 34: 234-240. 1947.
66a. Chilton, M.-D., Drummond, M. H., Merlo, D. J., et al. Stable incorporation of plasmid DNA into higher plant cells: the molecular basis of crown gall tumorigenesis. Cell 11:263-271. 1977.
67. Braun, A. C. Conditioning of the host cell as a factor in the transformation process in crown gall. Growth 16:65-74. 1952.
68. Braun, A. C., and Mandle, R. J. Studies on the inactivation of the tumor-inducing principle in crown gall. Growth 12:255-269. 1948.
69. Black, L. M. Plant tumors of viral origin. Progr. Exptl. Tumor Res. 15:110-137. 1972.
70. Smith, H. H. Plant genetic tumors. Progr. Exptl. Tumor Res. 15:138-164. 1972.
71. Borek, C., and Sachs, L. *In vitro* cell transformation by X-irradiation. Nature 210:276-278. 1966.
72. Berwald, Y., and Sachs, L. *In vitro* transformation of normal cells to tumor cells by carcinogenic hydrocarbons. J. Natl. Cancer Inst. 35:641-661. 1965.
73. Todaro, G. J., and Green, H. Cell growth and the initiation of transformation by SV40. Proc. Natl. Acad. Sci. USA 55:302-308. 1966.
74. Braun, A. C., and Wood, H. N. On the activation of certain essential biosynthetic systems in cells of *Vinca rosea* L. Proc. Natl. Acad. Sci. USA 48:1776-1782. 1962.
75. Wood, H. N., and Braun, A. C. Studies on the regulation of certain essential biosynthetic systems in normal and crown-gall tumor cells. Proc. Natl. Acad. Sci. USA

47:1907-1913. 1961.
76. Wood, H. N., and Braun, A. C. Studies on the net uptake of solutes by normal and crown-gall tumor cells. Proc. Natl. Acad. Sci. USA 54:1532-1538. 1965.
77. Foster, D. O., and Pardee, A. B. Transport of amino acids by confluent and nonconfluent 3T3 and polyoma virus-transformed 3T3 cells growing on glass cover slips. J. Biol. Chem. 244:2675-2681. 1969.
78. Hatanaka, M., and Hanafusa, H. Analysis of a functional change in membrane in the process of cell transformation by Rous sarcoma virus; alteration in the characteristics of sugar transport. Virology 41:647-652. 1970.
79. Isselbacher, K. J. Increased uptake of amino acids and 2-deoxy-D-glucose by virus-transformed cells in culture. Proc. Natl. Acad. Sci. USA 69:585-589. 1972.
80. Oshiro, Y., and DiPaolo, J. A. Changes in the uptake of 2-deoxy-D-glucose in Balb/3T3 cells chemically transformed in culture. J. Cell. Physiol. 83:193-202. 1974.
81. Balk, S. D., Whitfield, J. F., Youdale, T., and Braun, A. C. Roles of calcium, serum, plasma, and folic acid in the control of proliferation of normal and Rous sarcoma virus-infected chicken fibroblasts. Proc. Natl. Acad. Sci. USA 70:675-679. 1973.
82. Dulbecco, R., and Elkington, J. Induction of growth in resting fibroblastic cell cultures by $Ca^{++}$. Proc. Natl. Acad. Sci. USA 72:1584-1588. 1975.
83. Whitfield, J. F., MacManus, J. P., Rixon, R. H., et al. The positive control of cell proliferation by the interplay of calcium ions and cyclic nucleotides; a review. In Vitro 12:1-18. 1976.
84. Swierenga, S. H. H., Whitfield, J. F., and Gillan, D. J. Alteration by malignant transformation of the calcium requirements for cell proliferation in vitro. J. Natl. Cancer Inst. 57:125-129. 1976.
85. Boynton, A. L., and Whitfield, J. F. Different calcium requirements for proliferation of conditionally and unconditionally tumorigenic mouse cells. Proc. Natl. Acad. Sci. USA 73:1651-1654. 1976.
86. Mitchell, R. S., Elgas, R. J., and Balk, S. D. Proliferation of Rous sarcoma virus-infected, but not of normal, chicken fibroblasts in oxygen-enriched environment: preliminary report. Proc. Natl. Acad. Sci. USA 73: 1265-1268. 1976.
87. Watterson, D. M., van Eldik, L. J., Smith, R. E., et al. Calcium-dependent regulatory protein of cyclic nucleotide metabolism in normal and transformed chicken embryo fibroblasts. Proc. Natl. Acad. Sci. USA 73:2711-2715.

1976.
88. Rubin, H., and Koide, T. Mutual potentiation by magnesium and calcium of growth in animal cells. Proc. Natl. Acad. Sci. USA 73:168-172. 1976.
89. Paul, D. Quiescent SV40 virus transformed 3T3 cells in culture. Biochem. Biophys. Res. Commun. 53:745-753. 1973.
90. Pardee, A. B. A restriction point for control of normal animal cell proliferation. Proc. Natl. Acad. Sci. USA 71:1286-1290. 1974.
91. Fischer, B. Die experimentelle Erzeugung atypischer Epithelwucherungen und die Entstehung bösartiger Geschwulste. Münch. Med. Wchnschr. 53:2041-2047. 1906.
92. Rubin, H. Overgrowth stimulating factor released from Rous sarcoma cells. Science 167:1271-1272. 1970.
93. Coman, D. R. Decreased mutual adhesiveness, a property of cells from squamous cell carcinomas. Cancer Res. 4:625-629. 1944.
94. Burger, M. M. A difference in the architecture of the surface membrane of normal and virally transformed cells. Proc. Natl. Acad. Sci. USA 62:994-1001. 1969.
95. Burger, M. M. Surface changes in transformed cells detected by lectins. Federation Proc. 32:91-101. 1973.
96. Burger, M. M., and Noonan, K. D. Restoration of normal growth by covering of agglutinin sites on tumour cell surface. Nature 228:512-515. 1970.
97. Noonan, K. D., Renger, H. C., Basilico, C., et al. Surface changes in temperature-sensitive simian virus 40-transformed cells. Proc. Natl. Acad. Sci. USA 70:347-349. 1973.
98. Nicolson, G. L. Difference in topology of normal and tumour cell membranes shown by different surface distributions of ferritin-conjugated concanavalin A. Nature New Biol. 233:244-246. 1971.
99. Ash, J. F., Vogt, P. K., and Singer, S. J. Reversion from transformed to normal phenotype by inhibition of protein synthesis in rat kidney cells infected with a temperature-sensitive mutant of Rous sarcoma virus. Proc. Natl. Acad. Sci. USA 73:3603-3607. 1976.
100. Cuatrecasas, P., and Tell, G. P. E. Insulin-like activity of concanavalin A and wheat germ agglutinin -- direct interactions with insulin receptors. Proc. Natl. Acad. Sci. USA 70:485-489. 1973.
101. Holley, R. W. A unifying hypothesis concerning the nature of malignant growth. Proc. Natl. Acad. Sci. USA 69:2840-2841. 1972.
102. Ossowski, L., Unkeless, J. C., Tobia, A., et al.

An enzymatic function associated with transformation of fibroblasts by oncogenic viruses. II. Mammalian fibroblast cultures transformed by DNA and RNA tumor viruses. J. Exptl. Med. 137:112-126. 1973.

103. Unkeless, J. C., Tobia, A., Ossowski, L., et al. An enzymatic function associated with transformation of fibroblasts by oncogenic viruses. I. Chick embryo fibroblast cultures transformed by avian RNA tumor viruses. J. Exptl. Med. 137:85-111. 1973.

104. Schnebli, H. P., and Burger, M. M. Selective inhibition of growth of transformed cells by protease inhibitors. Proc. Natl. Acad. Sci. USA 69:3825-3827. 1972.

105. Chou, I.-N., Black, P. H., and Roblin, R. O. Suppression of fibrinolysin T activity fails to restore density-dependent growth inhibition to SV3T3 cells. Nature 250:739-741. 1974.

106. Ossowski, L., Quigley, J. P., Kellerman, G. M., et al. Fibrinolysis associated with oncogenic transformation. J. Exptl. Med. 138:1056-1064. 1973.

107. Bürk, R. R. A factor from a transformed cell line that affects cell migration. Proc. Natl. Acad. Sci. USA 70:369-372. 1973.

108. Lipkin, G., and Knecht, M. E. A diffusible factor restoring contact inhibition of growth to malignant melanocytes. Proc. Natl. Acad. Sci. USA 71:849-853. 1974.

109. Jinks, J. L. Extrachromosomal Inheritance. 177 pp. Prentice-Hall, Englewood Cliffs, N.J., 1964.

110. Wilkie, D. The Cytoplasm in Heredity. 115 pp. Methuen, London, 1964.

111. Sonneborn, T. M. Kappa particles and their bearing on host-parasite relations. Perspectives Virol. 2:5-17. 1961.

112. Jollos, V. Experimentelle Protistenstudien. I. Untersuchungen über Variabilität und Vererbung bei Infusorien. Arch. Protistenkunde 43:1-222. 1921.

113. Beale, G. H. The role of the cytoplasm in antigen determination in Paramecium aurelia. Proc. Roy. Soc. (London), Ser. B, 148:308-314. 1958.

114. Beale, G. H. The Genetics of Paramecium aurelia. The University Press, Cambridge [Eng.], 1954.

115. Sonneborn, T. M., Does preformed cell structure play an essential role in cell heredity? in The Nature of Biological Diversity (J. M. Allen, ed.) p. 165-221. McGraw-Hill, New York, 1963.

116. Binns, A., and Meins, F., Jr. Habituation of tobacco pith cells for factors promoting cell division is heritable and potentially reversible. Proc. Natl.

Acad. Sci. USA 70:2660-2662. 1973. See also Meins, F., Jr., and Binns, A. Epigenetic variation of cultured somatic cells: evidence for gradual changes in the requirement for factors promoting cell division. Proc. Natl. Acad. Sci. USA 74:2928-2932. 1977.

117. Lutz, A. Morphogenetic aptitudes of tissue cultures of unicellular origin. in Colloq. Internat. Centre Nat. Recherche Sci. (Paris), No. 193, Les Cultures de Tissus de Plantes. p. 163-168. Centre National de la Recherche Scientifique, Paris, 1971.

118. Braun, A. C. A demonstration of the recovery of the crown-gall tumor cell with the use of complex tumors of single-cell origin. Proc. Natl. Acad. Sci. USA 45:932-938. 1959.

119. Braun, A. C., and Wood, H. N. Suppression of the neoplastic state with the acquisition of specialized functions in cells, tissues, and organs of crown gall teratomas of tobacco. Proc. Natl. Acad. Sci. USA 73: 496-500. 1976.

120. Turgeon, R., Wood, H. N., and Braun, A. C. Studies on the recovery of crown gall tumor cells. Proc. Natl. Acad. Sci. USA 73:3562-3564. 1976.

120a. Sacristán, M. D., and Melchers, G. Regeneration of plants from "habituated" and "Agrobacterium-transformed" single-cell clones of tobacco. Molec. Gen. Genet. 152:111-117. 1977.

121. Kleinsmith, L. J., and Pierce, G. B., Jr. Multipotentiality of single embryonal carcinoma cells. Cancer Res. 24:1544-1551. 1964.

122. Illmensee, K., and Mintz, B. Totipotency and normal differentiation of single teratocarcinoma cells cloned by injection into blastocysts. Proc. Natl. Acad. Sci. USA 73:549-553. 1976.

123. Pierce, G. B., and Wallace, C. Differentiation of malignant to benign cells. Cancer Res. 31:127-134. 1971.

124. McKinnell, R. G., Deggins, B. A., and Labat, D. D. Transplantation of pluripotential nuclei from triploid frog tumors. Science 165:394-396. 1969. See also McKinnell, R. G., Steven, L. M., Jr., and Labat, D. D. Frog renal tumors are composed of stroma, vascular elements and epithelial cells: what type nucleus programs for tadpoles with the cloning procedure? in Progress in Differentiation Research (N. Müller-Bérat, et al., eds.) p. 319-330. North-Holland Publ. Co., Amsterdam, The Netherlands, 1976.

125. Cushing, H., and Wolbach, S. B. The transformation of a malignant paravertebral sympathicoblastoma into a

benign ganglioneuroma. Am. J. Pathol. 3:203-216. 1927.
126. Dyke, P. C., and Mulkey, D. A. Maturation of ganglioneuroblastoma to ganglioneuroma. Cancer 20:1343-1349. 1967.
127. Visfeldt, J. Transformation of sympathicoblastoma into ganglioneuroma. With a case report. Acta Pathol. Microbiol. Scand. 58:414-428. 1963.
128. Everson, T. C., and Cole, W. H. Spontaneous Regression of Cancer. 560 pp. W. B. Saunders, Philadelphia and London, 1966.
129. Kimhi, Y., Palfrey, C., Spector, I., et al. Maturation of neuroblastoma cells in the presence of dimethylsulfoxide. Proc. Natl. Acad. Sci. USA 73:462-466. 1976.
130. Friend, C., Scher, W., Holland, J. G., et al. Hemoglobin synthesis in murine virus-induced leukemic cells in vitro: stimulation of erythroid differentiation by dimethyl sulfoxide. Proc. Natl. Acad. Sci. USA 68: 378-382. 1971.
131. Fibach, E., Landau, T., and Sachs, L. Normal differentiation of myeloid leukaemic cells induced by a differentiation-inducing protein. Nature New Biol. 237:276-278. 1972.
132. Metcalf, D., Bradley, T. R., and Robinson, W. Analysis of colonies developing in vitro from mouse bone marrow cells stimulated by kidney feeder layers or leukemic serum. J. Cellular Physiol. 69:93-108. 1967.
133. Worton, R. G., McCulloch, E. A., and Till, J. E. Physical separation of hemopoietic stem cells from cells forming colonies in culture. J. Cellular Physiol. 74:171-182. 1969.
134. Basile, D. V., Wood, H. N., and Braun, A. C. Programming of cells for death under defined experimental conditions: relevance to the tumor problem. Proc. Natl. Acad. Sci. USA 70:3055-3059. 1973.
135. Wahn, H. L., Lightbody, L. E., Tchen, T. T., et al. Induction of neural differentiation in cultures of amphibian undetermined presumptive epidermis by cyclic AMP derivatives. Science 188:366-369. 1975.
136. Rous, P. Surmise and fact on the nature of cancer. Nature 183:1357-1361. 1959.
137. Kark, W. A Synopsis of Cancer. Genesis and Biology. 280 pp. John Wright and Sons, Ltd., Bristol, 1966.
138. Bayreuther, K. Chromosomes in primary neoplastic growth. Nature 186:6-9. 1960.
139. DiBerardino, M. A., King, T. J., and McKinnell, R. G. Chromosome studies of a frog renal adenocarcinoma

line carried by serial intraocular transplantation. J. Natl. Cancer Inst. 31:769-789. 1963.
140. Dunn, G. R., and Stevens, L. C. Determination of sex of teratomas derived from early mouse embryos. J. Natl. Cancer Inst. 44:99-105. 1970.
141. Levan, A. Some current problems of cancer cytogenetics. Hereditas 57:343-355. 1967.
142. Nowell, P. C., and Hungerford, D. A. Chromosome studies in human leukemia. II. Chronic granulocytic leukemia. J. Natl. Cancer Inst. 27:1013-1035. 1961.
143. Rowley, J. D. A new consistent chromosomal abnormality in chronic myelogenous leukaemia identified by quinacrine fluorescence and Giemsa staining. Nature 243:290-293. 1973.
144. Todaro, G. J., Green, H., and Swift, M. R. Susceptibility of human diploid fibroblast strains to transformation by SV40 virus. Science 153:1252-1254. 1966.
145. Rabinowitz, Z., and Sachs, L. Reversion of properties in cells transformed by polyoma virus. Nature 220:1203-1206. 1968.
146. Bloch-Shtacher, N., Rabinowitz, Z., and Sachs, L. Chromosomal mechanism for the induction of reversion in transformed cells. Intern. J. Cancer 9:632-640. 1972.
147. Rabinowitz, Z., and Sachs, L. Control of the reversion of properties in transformed cells. Nature 225:136-139. 1970.
148. Hitotsumachi, S., Rabinowitz, Z., and Sachs, L. Chromosomal control of reversion in transformed cells. Nature 231:511-514. 1971.
149. Cho, H. Y., Cutchins, E. C., Rhim, J. S., et al. Revertants of human cells transformed by murine sarcoma virus. Science 194:951-953. 1976.
150. Harris, H., Miller, O. J., Klein, G., et al. Suppression of malignancy by cell fusion. Nature 223:363-368. 1969.
151. Wiener, F., Klein, G., and Harris, H. The analysis of malignancy by cell fusion. III. Hybrids between diploid fibroblasts and other tumour cells. J. Cell Sci. 8:681-692. 1971.
152. Gordon, M. A genetic concept for the origin of melanomas. Ann. New York Acad. Sci. 71:1213-1222. 1958.
153. Little, C. C. The genetics of cancer in mice. Biol. Rev. Cambridge Phil. Soc. 22:315-343. 1947.
154. Carlson, P. S., Smith, H. H., and Dearing, R. D. Parasexual interspecific plant hybridization. Proc. Natl. Acad. Sci. USA 69:2292-2294. 1972. See also Smith, H. H., Kao, K. N., and Combatti, N. C.

Interspecific hybridization by protoplast fusion in *Nicotiana*. J. Heredity 67:123-128. 1976.
155. Nichols, W. W., Levan, A., and Heneen, W. K. Studies on the role of viruses in somatic mutation. Hereditas 57:365-368. 1967.
156. Macpherson, I. Reversion in hamster cells transformed by Rous sarcoma virus. Science 148:1731-1733. 1965.
157. Knudson, A. G., Jr. Mutation and cancer: statistical study of retinoblastoma. Proc. Natl. Acad. Sci. USA 68:820-823. 1971.
158. Gross, L. Serial cell-free passage of a radiation-activated mouse leukemia agent. Proc. Soc. Exptl. Biol. Med. 100:102-105. 1959.
159. Lieberman, M., and Kaplan, H. S. Leukemogenic activity of filtrates from radiation-induced lymphoid tumors of mice. Science 130:387-388. 1959.
160. U.S. National Program for the Conquest of Cancer. Report of the National Panel of Consultants on the Conquest of Cancer. Authorized by S. Res. 376. Prepared for the Committee on Labor and Public Welfare, U.S. Senate, Nov. 1970. Report No. 91-1402. 150 pp. Washington, D.C., 1971. (See page 100)
161. Setlow, R. B., Regan, J. D., German, J., et al. Evidence that xeroderma pigmentosum cells do not perform the first step in the repair of ultraviolet damage to their DNA. Proc. Natl. Acad. Sci. USA 64:1035-1041. 1969.
162. Ames, B. N., Durston, W. E., Yamasaki, E., et al. Carcinogens are mutagens: a simple test system combining liver homogenates for activation and bacteria for detection. Proc. Natl. Acad. Sci. USA 70:2281-2285. 1973.
163. Rubin, H. Carcinogenicity tests. Science 191:241. 1976.
164. Sivak, A. The Ames assay. Science 193:272-274. 1976.
165. Berwald, Y., and Sachs, L. *In vitro* cell transformation with chemical carcinogens. Nature 200:1182-1184. 1963.
166. Huberman, E., and Sachs, L. Cell susceptibility to transformation and cytotoxicity by the carcinogenic hydrocarbon benzo[A]pyrene. Proc. Natl. Acad. Sci. USA 56:1123-1129. 1966.
167. Mondal, S., and Heidelberger, C. *In vitro* malignant transformation by methylcholanthrene of the progeny of single cells derived from C3H mouse prostate. Proc. Natl. Acad. Sci. USA 65:219-225. 1970.
168. Huberman, E., Mager, R., and Sachs, L. Mutagenesis and transformation of normal cells by chemical carcinogens. Nature 264:360-361. 1976.

169. Ursprung, H. Fragmentierungs- und Bestrahlungsversuche zur Bestimmung von Determinationszustand und Anlageplan der Genitalscheiben von _Drosophila melanogaster_. Arch. Entwicklungsmech. Organ. _151_:504-558. 1959.
170. Nöthiger, R. Differenzierungsleistungen in Kombinaten, hergestellt aus Imaginalscheiben verschiedener Arten, Geschlechter und Körpersegmente von _Drosophila_. Arch. Entwicklungsmech. Organ. _155_:269-301. 1964.
171. Hadorn, E., Bertani, G., and Gallera, J. Regulationsfähigkeit und Feltorganisation der männlichen Genital-Imaginalscheibe von _Drosophila melanogaster_. Arch. Entwicklungsmech. Organ. _144_:31-70. 1949.
172. Wolff, E., and Ginglinger, A. Sur la production expérimentale d'intersexués par l'injection de folliculine à l'embryon de poulet. C. r. Acad. Sci., Paris _200_: 2118-2120. 1935.
173. Rous, P. Opening remarks. Am. Cancer Soc. Symp., "The Possible Role of Viruses in Cancer." Cancer Res. _20_: 672-676. 1960.
174. Stewart, S. E., Eddy, B. E., and Borgese, N. Neoplasms in mice inoculated with a tumor agent carried in tissue culture. J. Natl. Cancer Inst. _20_:1223-1243. 1958.
175. Naegele, R. F., Granoff, A., and Darlington, R. W. The presence of the Lucké herpesvirus genome in induced tadpole tumors and its oncogenicity: Koch-Henle postulates fulfilled. Proc. Natl. Acad. Sci. USA _71_:830-834. 1974.
176. Burmeister, B. R. Viruses of the leukosis/sarcoma group. _in_ Poultry Diseases and World Economy (R. F. Gordon and B. M. Freedman, eds.) p. 135-152. British Poultry Science, Edinburgh, 1971.
177. Klein, G. Herpesviruses and oncogenesis. Proc. Natl. Acad. Sci. USA _69_:1056-1064. 1972.
178. Kufe, D., Magrath, I. T., Ziegler, J. L., et al. Burkitt's tumors contain particles encapsulating RNA-instructed DNA polymerase and high molecular weight virus-related RNA. Proc. Natl. Acad. Sci. USA _70_: 737-741. 1973.
179. Sambrook, J., Westphal, H., Srinivasan, P. R., et al. The integrated state of viral DNA in SV40-transformed cells. Proc. Natl. Acad. Sci. USA _60_:1288-1295. 1968.
180. Benjamin, T. L. Virus-specific RNA in cells productively infected or transformed by polyoma virus. J. Mol. Biol. _16_:359-373. 1966.
181. Fujinaga, K., and Green, M. The mechanism of viral carcinogenesis by DNA mammalian viruses: viral-specific

RNA in polyribosomes of adenovirus tumor and transformed cells. Proc. Natl. Acad. Sci. USA 55:1567-1574. 1966.

182. Watkins, J. F., and Dulbecco, R. Production of SV40 virus in heterokaryons of transformed and susceptible cells. Proc. Natl. Acad. Sci. USA 58:1396-1403. 1967.

183. Koprowski, H., Jensen, F. C., and Steplewski, Z. Activation of production of infectious tumor virus SV40 in heterokaryon cultures. Proc. Natl. Acad. Sci. USA 58:127-133. 1967.

184. Martin, R. G., and Chou, J. Y. Simian virus 40 functions required for the establishment and maintenance of malignant transformation. J. Virology 15:599-612. 1975.

184a. Tegtmeyer, P. Function of simian virus 40 gene A in transforming infection. J. Virology 15:613-618. 1975.

184b. Brugge, J. S., and Butel, J. S. Role of simian virus 40 gene A function in maintenance of transformation. J. Virology 15:619-635. 1975.

184c. Osborn, M., and Weber, K. Simian virus 40 gene A function and maintenance of transformation. J. Virology 15:636-644. 1975.

185. Graessmann, M., and Graessmann, A. "Early" simian-virus-40-specific RNA contains information for tumor antigen formation and chromatin replication. Proc. Natl. Acad. Sci. USA 73:366-370. 1976.

186. Basilico, C., and Zouzias, D. Regulation of viral transcription and tumor antigen expression in cells transformed by simian virus 40. Proc. Natl. Acad. Sci. USA 73:1931-1935. 1976.

187. Ahmad-Zadeh, C., Allet, B., Greenblatt, J., et al. Two forms of simian-virus-40-specific T-antigen in abortive and lytic infection. Proc. Natl. Acad. Sci. USA 73:1097-1101. 1976.

188. Pollack, R. E., Green, H., and Todaro, G. J. Growth control in cultured cells: selection of sublines with increased sensitivity to contact inhibition and decreased tumor-producing ability. Proc. Natl. Acad. Sci. USA 60:126-133. 1968.

189. Sjögren, H. O., Hellström, I., and Klein, G. Transplantation of polyoma virus-induced tumors in mice. Cancer Res. 21:329-337. 1961.

190. Habel, K. Resistance of polyoma immune animals to transplanted polyoma tumors. Proc. Soc. Exptl. Biol. Med. 106:722-725. 1961.

191. Billeter, M. A., Parsons, J. T., and Coffin, J. M. The nucleotide sequence complexity of avian tumor virus

RNA. Proc. Natl. Acad. Sci. USA 71:3560-3564. 1974.
192. Beemon, K., Duesberg, P., and Vogt, P. Evidence for crossing-over between avian tumor viruses based on analysis of viral RNAs. Proc. Natl. Acad. Sci. USA 71:4254-4258. 1974.
193. Baltimore, D. Tumor viruses: 1974. Cold Spring Harbor Symp. Quant. Biol. 39:1187-1200. 1975.
194. Stehelin, D., Guntaka, R. V., Varmus, H. E., et al. Purification of DNA complementary to nucleotide sequences required for neoplastic transformation of fibroblasts by avian sarcoma viruses. J. Mol. Biol. 101:349-365. 1976.
195. Wang, L.-H., Duesberg, P. H., Kawai, S., et al. Location of envelope-specific and sarcoma-specific oligonucleotides on RNA of Schmidt-Ruppin Rous sarcoma virus. Proc. Natl. Acad. Sci. USA 73:447-451. 1976.
196. Sloan-Kettering Institute, Report. [Hardy, W. D., Jr., et al.] Horizontal transmission of feline leukemia virus in cats. Memorial Sloan-Kettering Cancer Center: Clinical Bull. 2:31-32. 1972.
197. Bittner, J. J. The milk-influence of breast tumors in mice. Science 95:462-463. 1942.
198. Lowy, D. R., Rowe, W. P., Teich, N., et al. Murine leukemia virus: high-frequency activation in vitro by 5-iododeoxyuridine and 5-bromodeoxyuridine. Science 174:155-156. 1971.
199. Aaronson, S. A., Todaro, G. J., and Scolnick, E. M. Induction of murine C-type viruses from clonal lines of virus-free BALB/3T3 cells. Science 174:157-159. 1971.
200. Huebner, R. J., and Todaro, G. J. Oncogenes of RNA tumor viruses as determinants of cancer. Proc. Natl. Acad. Sci. USA 64:1087-1094. 1969.
201. Todaro, G. J., and Huebner, R. J. The viral oncogene hypothesis: new evidence. Proc. Natl. Acad. Sci. USA 69:1009-1015. 1972.
202. Baxt, W., Yates, J. W., Wallace, H. J., Jr., et al. Leukemia-specific DNA sequences in leukocytes of the leukemic member of identical twins. Proc. Natl. Acad. Sci. USA 70:2629-2632. 1973.
203. Reitz, M. S., Miller, N. R., Wong-Staal, F., et al. Primate type-C virus nucleic acid sequences (woolly monkey and baboon types) in tissues from a patient with acute myelogenous leukemia and in viruses isolated from cultured cells of the same patient. Proc. Natl. Acad. Sci. USA 73:2113-2117. 1976.
204. Baltimore, D. RNA-dependent DNA polymerase in virions

of RNA tumour viruses. Nature 226:1209-1211. 1970.
205. Temin, H. M., and Mizutani, S. RNA-dependent DNA polymerase in virions of Rous sarcoma virus. Nature 226:1211-1213. 1970.
206. Varmus, H. E., Vogt, P. K., and Bishop, J. M. Integration of deoxyribonucleic acid specific for Rous sarcoma virus after infection of permissive and nonpermissive hosts. Proc. Natl. Acad. Sci. USA 70:3067-3071. 1973.
207. Temin, H. M. The protovirus hypothesis: speculations on the significance of RNA-directed DNA synthesis for normal development and for carcinogenesis. J. Natl. Cancer Inst. 46:III-VII. 1971.
208. Stephenson, J. R., Reynolds, R. K., and Aaronson, S. A. Characterization of morphologic revertants of murine and avian sarcoma virus-transformed cells. J. Virology 11:218-222. 1973.
209. Toyoshima, K., and Vogt, P. K. Temperature sensitive mutants of an avian sarcoma virus. Virology 39:930-931. 1969.
210. Wickus, G. G., and Robbins, P. W. Plasma membrane proteins of normal and Rous sarcoma virus-transformed chick-embryo fibroblasts. Nature New Biol. 245:65-67. 1973.
211. Warren, L., Critchley, D., and Macpherson, I. Surface glycoproteins and glycolipids of chicken embryo cells transformed by a temperature-sensitive mutant of Rous sarcoma virus. Nature 235:275-277. 1972.
212. Deng, C.-T., Boettiger, D., Macpherson, I., et al. The persistence and expression of virus-specific DNA in revertants of Rous sarcoma virus-transformed BHK-21 cells. Virology 62:512-521. 1974.
213. Frankel, A. E., Haapala, D. K., Neubauer, R. L., et al. Elimination of the sarcoma genome from murine sarcoma virus transformed cat cells. Science 191:1264-1266. 1976.
214. Todaro, G. J., Lazar, G. K., and Green, H. The initiation of cell division in a contact-inhibited mammalian cell line. J. Cellular Comp. Physiol. 66:325-334. 1965.
215. Holley, R. W., and Kiernan, J. A. "Contact inhibition" of cell division in 3T3 cells. Proc. Natl. Acad. Sci. USA 60:300-304. 1968.
216. Holley, R. W., and Kiernan, J. A. Control of the initiation of DNA synthesis in 3T3 cells: serum factors. Proc. Natl. Acad. Sci. USA 71:2908-2911. 1974.
217. Holley, R. W. Control of growth of mammalian cells in cell culture. Nature 258:487-490. 1975.

218. Temin, H. M. Studies on carcinogenesis by avian sarcoma viruses. VI. Differential multiplication of uninfected and of converted cells in response to insulin. J. Cellular Physiol. 69:377-384. 1967.
219. Temin, H. M. Control by factors in serum of multiplication of uninfected cells and cells infected and converted by avian sarcoma viruses. in Growth Regulating Substances for Animal Cells in Culture (V. Defendi and M. Stoker, eds.) p. 103-116. Wistar Inst. Press, Philadelphia, 1967.
220. Stoker, M. Abortive transformation by polyoma virus. Nature 218:234-238. 1968.
221. Stoker, M., O'Neill, C., Berryman, S., et al. Anchorage and growth regulation in normal and virus-transformed cells. Intern. J. Cancer 3:683-693. 1968.
222. Pollack, R., Risser, R., Conlon, S., et al. Production of plasminogen activator and colonial growth in semi-solid medium are in vitro correlates of tumorigenicity in the immune-deficient nude mouse. in Proteases and Biological Control (Reich, E., Rifkin, D. B., and Shaw, E., eds.) Vol. 2, p. 885-899. Cold Spring Harbor Laboratory, New York, 1975.
223. Abbott, J., and Holtzer, H. The loss of phenotypic traits by differentiated cells, V. The effect of 5-bromodeoxyuridine on cloned chondrocytes. Proc. Natl. Acad. Sci. USA 59:1144-1151. 1968.
224. Bischoff, R., and Holtzer, H. Inhibition of hyaluronic acid synthesis by BUdR in cultures of chick amnion cells. Anat. Record 160:317. 1968.
225. Bischoff, R., and Holtzer, H. Inhibition of myoblast fusion after one round of DNA synthesis in 5-bromodeoxyuridine. J. Cell Biol. 44:134-150. 1970.
226. Coleman, A. W., Kunkel, D., Werener, I., et al. Cellular differentiation in vitro: perturbation by halogenated deoxyribonucleosides. J. Cell Biol. 39:27a. 1968.
227. Coleman, J. R., Coleman, A. W., and Hartline, E. J. H. A clonal study of the reversible inhibition of muscle differentiation by the halogenated thymidine analog 5-bromodeoxyuridine. Develop. Biol. 19:527-548. 1969.
228. Lasher, R., and Cahn, R. D. The effects of 5-bromodeoxyuridine on the differentiation of chondrocytes *in vitro*. Develop. Biol. 19:415-435. 1969.
229. Stellwagen, R. H., and Tomkins, G. M. Preferential inhibition by 5-bromodeoxyuridine of the synthesis of tyrosine aminotransferase in hepatoma cell cultures. J. Mol. Biol. 56:167-182. 1971.
230. Silagi, S., and Bruce, S. A. Suppression of malignancy

and differentiation in melanotic melanoma cells. Proc. Natl. Acad. Sci. USA 66:72-78. 1970.
231. Silagi, S., Beju, D., Wrathall, J., et al. Tumorigenicity, immunogenicity, and virus production in mouse melanoma cells treated with 5-bromodeoxyuridine. Proc. Natl. Acad. Sci. USA 69:3443-3447. 1972.
232. Christman, J. K., Silagi, S., Newcomb, E. W., et al. Correlated suppression by 5-bromodeoxyuridine of tumorigenicity and plasminogen activator in mouse melanoma cells. Proc. Natl. Acad. Sci. USA 72:47-50. 1975.
233. Wigler, M., and Weinstein, I. B. Tumour promotor induces plasminogen activator. Nature 259:232-233. 1976.
234. Silagi, S. Effects of 5-bromodeoxyuridine on tumorigenicity, immunogenicity, virus production, plasminogen activator, and melanogenesis of mouse melanoma cells. Intern. Rev. Cytol. 45:65-111. 1976.
235. Swann, M. M. The control of cell division: a review. II. Special mechanisms. Cancer Res. 18:1118-1160. 1958.
236. Boone, C. W. Malignant hemangioendotheliomas produced by subcutaneous inoculation of Balb/3T3 cells attached to glass beads. Science 188:68-70. 1975.
237. Abelev, G. I., Perova, S. D., Khramkova, N. I., et al. Embryonic serum alpha-globulin and its synthesis by transplantable mouse hepatomas. Biokhimiya 28:625-634. 1963.
238. Gold, P., and Freedman, S. O. Demonstration of tumor-specific antigens in human colonic carcinomata by immunological tolerance and absorption techniques. J. Exptl. Med. 121:439-462. 1965.
239. Gold, P., and Freedman, S. O. Specific carcinoembryonic antigens of the human digestive system. J. Exptl. Med. 122:467-481. 1965.
240. Gellhorn, A. Ectopic hormone production in cancer and its implication for basic research on abnormal growth. Advan. Internal Med. 15:299-316. 1969.
241. Lipsett, M. B., Odell, W. D., Rosenberg, L. E., et al. Humoral syndromes associated with nonendocrine tumors. Ann. Internal Med. 61:733-756. 1964.
242. Marks, L. J., Russfield, A. B., and Rosenbaum, D. L. Corticotropin-secreting carcinoma. J. Am. Med. Assoc. 183, No. 2:115-117. 1963.
243. Faiman, C., Colwell, J. A., Ryan, R. J., et al. Gonadotropin secretion from a bronchogenic carcinoma. Demonstration by radioimmunoassay. New England J. Med. 277:1395-1399. 1967.

244. Bullough, W. S., and Laurence, E. B. Tissue homeostasis in adult mammals. in Advances in Biology of Skin (W. Montagna and R. L. Dobson, eds.), Carcinogenesis, Vol. 7, p. 1-36. Pergamon Press, London and New York, 1966.

245. Goldberger, R. F. Autogenous regulation of gene expression. Science 183:810-816. 1974.

246. Cohen, G. N. Regulation of enzyme activity in microorganisms. Ann. Rev. Microbiol. 19:105-126. 1965.

247. Atkinson, D. E. Regulation of enzyme activity. Ann. Rev. Biochem. 35:85-124. 1966.

248. Allfrey, V. G., Faulkner, R., and Mirsky, A. E. Acetylation and methylation of histones and their possible role in the regulation of RNA synthesis. Proc. Natl. Acad. Sci. USA 51:786-794. 1964.

249. Allfrey, V. G., Littau, V. C., and Mirsky, A. E. On the role of histones in regulating ribonucleic acid synthesis in the cell nucleus. Proc. Natl. Acad. Sci. USA 49:414-421. 1963.

250. Stein, G. S., Spelsberg, T. C., and Kleinsmith, L. J. Nonhistone chromosomal proteins and gene regulation. Science 183:817-824. 1974.

251. Kleinsmith, L. J., Stein, J., and Stein, G. Dephosphorylation of nonhistone proteins specifically alters the pattern of gene transcription in reconstituted chromatin. Proc. Natl. Acad. Sci. USA 73:1174-1178. 1976.

252. Allfrey, V. G. Structural modifications of histones and their possible role in the regulation of ribonucleic acid synthesis. Canadian Cancer Res. Conf. 6:313-335. 1966.

253. Robertson, H. D., and Dickson, E. RNA processing and the control of gene expression. Brookhaven Symp. Biol. 26:240-266. 1974.

254. Miller, J. A., and Miller, E. C. Carcinogens occurring naturally in foods. Federation Proc. 35:1316-1321. 1976.

255. Sporn, M. B., Dunlop, N. M., Newton, D. L., et al. Prevention of chemical carcinogenesis by vitamin A and its synthetic analogs (retinoids). Federation Proc. 35:1332-1338. 1976.

256. Kinoshita, N., and Gelboin, H. V. Aryl hydrocarbon hydroxylase and polycyclic hydrocarbon tumorigenesis: effect of the enzyme inhibitor 7,8-benzoflavone on tumorigenesis and macromolecule binding. Proc. Natl. Acad. Sci. USA 69:824-828. 1972.

257. Weisburger, J. H., Yamamoto, R. S., Grantham, P. H.,

et al. Evidence that sulfate esters are key ultimate carcinogens from N-hydroxy-N-2-fluorenylacetamide. Proc. Am. Assoc. Cancer Res. 11:82, Abst. 325. 1970.

258. Miller, J. A., and Miller, E. C. Chemical carcinogenesis: mechanisms and approaches to its control. J. Natl. Cancer Inst. 47:V-XIV. 1971.

259. Warburg, O. Versuche an überlebendem Carcinomgewebe. Biochem. Z. 142:317-333. 1923.

260. Anderson, N. G., and Coggin, J. H., Jr., eds. Proceedings of the First Conference and Workshop on Embryonic and Fetal Antigens in Cancer, May 24-26, 1971. Oak Ridge National Laboratory, Oak Ridge, Tennessee, 400 pp. U.S. AEC Conf-710527, [1971].

261. Powell, A. E., Sloss, A. M., Smith, R. N., et al. Specific responsiveness of leukocytes to soluble extracts of human tumors. Intern. J. Cancer 16:905-913. 1975.

262. Gross, R. L., Levin, A. G., Steel, C. M., et al. In vitro immunological studies on East African cancer patients. II. Increased sensitivity of blood lymphocytes from untreated Burkitt lymphoma patients to inhibition of spontaneous rosette formation. Intern. J. Cancer 15:132-138. 1975.

263. Folkman, J. Tumor angiogenesis: therapeutic implications. New England J. Med. 285:1182-1186. 1971.

264. Langer, R., Brem, H., Falterman, K., et al. Isolation of a cartilage factor that inhibits tumor neovascularization. Science 193:70-72. 1976.

265. Carter, S. K., and Kershner, L. M. What you should know about drugs vs. cancer. Pharmacy Times p. 56-62, 66. August 1975.

266. Bonadonna, G., Brusamolino, E., Valagussa, P., et al. Combination chemotherapy as an adjuvant treatment in operable breast cancer. New England J. Med. 294:405-410. 1976.

267. Broome, J. D. Evidence that the L-asparaginase activity of guinea pig serum is responsible for its antilymphoma effects. Nature 191:1114-1115. 1961.

268. Krim, M., ed., et al. International Workshop on Interferon in the Treatment of Cancer, March 31, April 1 and 2, 1975, New York. Part 1: Report; part 2: Report Summary and Excerpted Conclusions and Recommendations. 134 pp.; 18 pp. New York, 1975.

269. Finter, N. B., ed. Interferons and Interferon Inducers. rev. ed., 598 pp. American Elsevier Publ. Co., New York, 1973.

270. Forscher, B. K., and Houck, J. C., eds. Chalones: concepts and current researches. 233 pp. National

Cancer Institute monograph 38. DHEW Publication No. (NIH) 73-425. National Cancer Institute, Bethesda, Md., 1973.

271. Verly, W. G., Deschamps, Y., Pushpathadam, J., et al. The hepatic chalone. I. Assay method for the hormone and purification of the rabbit liver chalone. Canadian J. Biochem. 49:1376-1383. 1971.

272. Gonzalez, R., and Verly, W. G. Isolation of an inhibitor of DNA synthesis specific for normal and malignant mammary cells. Proc. Natl. Acad. Sci. USA 73:2196-2200. 1976.

273. Hondius Boldingh, W., and Laurence, E. B. Extraction, purification and preliminary characterisation of the epidermal chalone: a tissue specific mitotic inhibitor obtained from vertebrate skin. European J. Biochem. 5:191-198. 1968.

274. Mohr, U., Althoff, J., Kinzel, V., et al. Melanoma regression induced by "chalone": a new tumour inhibiting principle acting in vivo. Nature 220:138-139. 1968.

275. Bullough, W. S., and Laurence, E. B. Control of mitosis in mouse and hamster melanomata by means of the melanocyte chalone. European J. Cancer 4:607-615. 1968.

276. Rytömaa, T., and Kiviniemi, K. Control of DNA duplication in rat chloroleukaemia by means of the granulocytic chalone. European J. Cancer 4:595-606. 1968.

276a. Rytömaa, T., and Kiviniemi, K. Chloroma regression induced by the granulocytic chalone. Nature 222:995-996. 1969.

277. Hellström, I., Hellström, K. E., Bill, A. H., et al. Studies on cellular immunity to human neuroblastoma cells. Intern. J. Cancer 6:172-188. 1970.

278. Kitagawa, M., Hamaoka, T., Takatsu, K., et al. Disturbance of immune surveillance in tumor-bearing host. GANN Monograph 16:45-52. 1974.

279. Prehn, R. T., and Lappé, M. A. An immunostimulation theory of tumor development. Transplantation Rev. 7:26-54. 1971.

280. Mathé, G., Halle-Pannenko, O., Bourut, C., et al. The use of systemic immunity adjuvants in the prophylaxis or therapy of cancer. in The Role of Immunological Factors in Viral and Oncogenic Processes (R. F. Beers, Jr., R. C. Tilghman, and E. G. Bassett, eds.) p. 85-102. The Johns Hopkins University Press, Baltimore, 1974.

281. Sparks, F. C., Silverstein, M. J., Hunt, J. S., et al.

Experimental and clinical trials with BCG immunotherapy. in The Role of Immunological Factors in Viral and Oncogenic Processes (R. F. Beers, Jr., R. C. Tilghman, and E. G. Bassett, eds.) p. 103-120. The Johns Hopkins University Press, Baltimore, 1974

282. Zbar, B. Immunotherapy of guinea pig cancer with BCG. in The Role of Immunological Factors in Viral and Oncogenic Processes (R. F. Beers, Jr., R. C. Tilghman, and E. G. Bassett, eds.) p. 121-130. The Johns Hopkins University Press, Baltimore, 1974.

283. Halpern, B. N., ed. Corynebacterium parvum; Applications in Experimental and Clinical Oncology. 444 pp. Plenum Press, New York, 1975.

284. Good, R. A. Clinical implications of the data base concerning the tumor-host relationship. in Immunobiology of the Tumor-Host Relationship (R. T. Smith and M. Landy, eds.) p. 277-350. Academic Press, New York, 1975.

## SUGGESTED ADDITIONAL READING

Oberling, Charles. The Riddle of Cancer. Translated by William H. Woglom. 196 pp. Yale University Press, New Haven, 1944. This book is an interesting and popularly written account of the cancer problem which reflects the thinking of a prominent figure among European students of cancer in the late 1930s and early 1940s.

Huxley, Julian. Biological Aspects of Cancer. 156 pp. Harcourt, Brace and Co., New York, 1958. This eminent British biologist reviews, for the scientifically informed, many facts about cancer in the light of advances made in biology up to the 1950s.

Braun, Armin C. The Cancer Problem: A Critical Analysis and Modern Synthesis. 209 pp. Columbia University Press, New York, 1969. The author views cancer as a problem in development and attempts to document that thesis.

Foulds, Leslie. Neoplastic Development. Vols. 1-2. Academic Press, New York, 1969-1975. An authoritative account of cancer written largely for specialists.

Braun, Armin C. The Biology of Cancer. 169 pp. Addison-Wesley Publ. Co., Reading, Mass., 1974. A short account written not for specialists but rather for beginners who have acquired a background in the basic biological sciences. The present book is an expanded and more detailed documentation of the concepts developed by the author in The Biology of Cancer and in The Cancer Problem.

Süss, Rudolf; Kinzel, Volker; and Scribner, John D. Cancer: Experiments and Concepts. Translated from the German by J. D. Scribner. 285 pp. Springer-Verlag, New York and Heidelberg, 1973. An introduction to problems and concepts involved in cancer research.

LaFond, Richard E., Guest Editor. Cancer--The Outlaw Cell. Chemistry Vol. 50, No. 1, p. 1-56. Jan.-Feb., 1977. A series of articles on cancer written by specialists in a popular style, designed to be understood by nonspecialists.

Becker, Frederick F., Editor. Cancer--A Comprehensive Treatise. Vols. 1-5. Plenum Press, New York, 1975-1977. Articles written by specialists for specialists. The most comprehensive treatise of various aspects of experimental cancer research.

## ACKNOWLEDGMENTS

The author gratefully acknowledges permission granted by Columbia University Press for the reproduction here, in whole or in part, of Figures 3, 4, 5, 6, 10, 12, 13, and 14 which had previously been used by the author in his book entitled "The Cancer Problem," Columbia University press, 1969; to Addison-Wesley Publishing Co., Inc., for permission to reproduce here, in whole or in part, Figures 2, 4, 5, 6, 7, and 8, previously published in the author's book "The Biology of Cancer," Addison-Wesley Publishing Co., Inc., 1974. He also wishes to express his gratitude to Dr. James S. Henderson, Dr. Roy E. Albert, and to the late Dr. Ian Macpherson for providing original prints used in Figures 6, 22, and 17, respectively, in the present book; to Science for permission to use the illustration shown in Figure 1 of the article entitled "Reversion of Hamster Cells Transformed by Rous Sarcoma Virus," by Ian Macpherson, Science 148:1731-1733, 1965, Copyright 1965, American Association for the Advancement of Science; to Springer Verlag, Vienna, for permission to use my illustrations previously published as Figures 3, 4, and 6 in "Morphology and Physiology of Plant Tumors," Protoplasmatologia 10, H.5a, 93 pp., 1958; as well as to the National Cancer Institute, DHEW, for continued grant support of the author's experimental studies, some of which are described here. The author is also grateful to Dr. Edward B. Ilgren for reading and discussing with the author certain sections of the book and to Dr. Henry N. Wood for preparing the illustrations shown in the frontispiece. I am particularly indebted to Ms. Ella Jeanne Ross for invaluable assistance in preparing and editing the manuscript for publication.

## SUBJECT INDEX